Take Care

Communicating
in English with
U.S. Health Care
Workers

Take Care

Communicating in English with U.S. Health Care Workers

Nina Ito

California State University, Long Beach

Christopher Mefford

California State University, Long Beach
Coastline Community College

Ann Arbor
University of Michigan Press

Acknowledgments

The authors wish to thank the following people who helped us with our needs analysis and subsequent content.

Nancy Andrews, RN, Vendored Nurse, Regional Center of Orange County, California
Michelle Angie, RN, MSN, NP, Cleveland Clinic, Ohio
Jasmine Holloway, RN, MSN, Methodist Medical Center, Illinois
Lori Kananack, MA Linguistics, Cedars Sinai Hospital, California
Candice Kim, pre-nursing student, Long Beach City College, California
Sherry Koupai, RN, Los Angeles Community Hospital, Kaiser Permanente, California
Ann Nguyen, RN, Fountain Valley Regional Hospital, California
Binh Nguyen, RN, Laguna Woods Senior Center, California
Evelyn Roth, nursing student, California State University, Long Beach, California
Miki Ueki, BSN, Keio University Hospital, Japan
Yokkaichi Nursing and Medical Care University nursing students, Japan

The publisher wishes to acknowledge the role of Robyn Brinks Lockwood as the developmental editor and the voice talent of Melissa Baker-Young, Gabriela Beres, Jason Contrucci, Heidi Dailey, Pat Grimes, Scott Ham, Badria Jazairi, Marcia LaBrenz, Sheryl Leicher, Heather Newman, Karen Pitton, Debra Shafer, and Laurel Stroud.

Contents

To the Teacher

About This Textbook

Nurses and other health care workers have an inherent need to communicate. If they are not able to communicate successfully, their jobs may be in jeopardy and, worse, patients may suffer. Instructors who use this textbook are in a position to help nursing students, certified nursing assistants (CNAs), nurses, and other health care workers attain communicative competence by improving their vocabulary, communication strategies, and pronunciation.

A knowledge of the field of nursing is not required for instructors who use this textbook. The majority of the material is language-based, not industry-based. The terminology that is used, such as *symptom, medication,* and *procedure,* is easy to understand. Any medical vocabulary that appears is used in context.

In constructing the scope and sequence of this book, we surveyed a variety of working nurses to learn which areas of the job (e.g., giving instructions, shift changes, etc.) are most crucial in day-to-day nursing in terms of clear communication. We also asked which language features (e.g., pronunciation, vocabulary, etc.) seemed to be most problematic for health care workers whose first language is not English. We also reviewed current textbooks in the nursing industry that focus on interpersonal communication. In addition, individual nursing students who are not fluent speakers of English were shown sample material to solicit their feedback. Some material in this book was pilot-tested with classes of ESL student nurses. Finally, multiple RNs were consulted as to the authenticity of the language used.

Who Will Benefit from This Textbook?

In compiling and developing the material that would make up this textbook, we envisioned these individuals as the ones who would benefit the most:

- Nursing students enrolled in community college (e.g., pre-nursing courses or RN students who have a special class)
- ESL students enrolled in specific CNA or medical assistant classes
- ESL students enrolled in U.S. universities who are here to learn more about nursing or health care as profession (they may or may not already have a degree in their own countries)
- Nurses or health care workers who already work in a health care setting but who are not proficient in English and so may be taking an English course sponsored by the hospital or local health system

It is therefore generally assumed that students have some knowledge of common medical and health care terms, so the book does not attempt to teach medical terminology, except in the context of communicating effectively in a health care setting. The various Vocabulary sections in each unit can therefore be used as review or as a new lesson—whatever works best for your students.

Why a Communication Strategies–Based Book?

Other English for Nursing or Health Care textbooks tend to be more academic, focusing on the same vocabulary and themes that students learn in their other nursing classes. For example, there may be a reading about wound care, which includes vocabulary like *dressing, debridement,* or *non-stick pads.* Thus, students practice reading skills and learn vocabulary, but they do not develop the skills necessary for face-to-face communication.

The nature of this textbook, however, is to give students the tools to build, maintain, or repair interactions that take place in their health care training or on the job in a health care setting. Thus, students will be able to communicate about wound care, asking colleagues questions such as, *I wonder if you can show me how to clean this wound.* or, *Did you say we need 15 or 50 bandages?* Or, for example, to make sure their message is understood by the client by using a "confirmation check," such as *Are you following me?* or *Sorry, did you catch that?* This text was designed to provide students with a firm grasp of verbal and non-verbal communication strategies, which will result in more successful interactions.

This textbook will also help develop pragmatic competence by asking students to practice the formulaic phrases needed to get things done. There are many specific social situations such as apologizing, giving advice, or expressing condolences, when the appropriate register and use of English is necessary.

A Note about Specific Terminology

The nursing terminology used in the textbook may differ from what some students have heard elsewhere because terminology is always evolving. One term that health care workers will have heard is *patient*, but the newer term, *client,* has been used throughout this textbook (although both terms are on the audio CD). As for equipment, some may say *cath bag,* while others say *Foley bag.* Most adults are familiar with the abbreviation ER for Emergency Room; however, recently more medical centers are using the term ED for Emergency Department or even EC for Emergency Center. Students may substitute terms used in their own facilities or words they are more familiar with for terms in the textbook if they wish. Note also that a large number of abbreviations and acronyms appear in this textbook. To help students, we have used periods for abbreviations (where letters are said) except in the cases of RN, CNA, and ED.

Contents

Take Care consists of 12 units in five thematic parts (Communicating with Clients, Communicating with Colleagues, Client Information, Around the Facility, and Caring for Clients). The textbook can be used in a quarter- or semester-long course. Ideally, the units should be studied in order as some material is recycled. Each unit is divided into two parts, each of which consists of seven sections.

Sections

Listening to the Action/Listening for Language

The focal point of each listening item is a conversation using content from either the Vocabulary or Communication Strategy sections from the unit. Students are asked to listen for specific words or phrases. Depending on students' level or experience, the instructor may want to play only the first conversation and then check students' answers before continuing. Students only need to write the key phrase, not the entire sentence, in the blanks provided. After playing the entire track once and checking for understanding, the instructor can then play it again so that students can check their answers. It is not necessary to go into detail about each answer as an explanation is given later in the unit. These items are recorded on the audio CD packaged with the text.

Dialogue

The Dialogue, set in a hospital or skilled nursing facility, contains examples of vocabulary items and communication strategies from the unit. Students should read this dialogue and practice pronunciation (stress, rhythm, intonation, and segmentals) as they work with a partner or small group. They may not understand all the vocabulary initially but will have ample practice opportunities throughout the unit. Dialogues are not recorded on the audio CD.

Vocabulary

Ten to 30 health care–related lexical items are included in each Vocabulary section. The students will be familiar with many of the individual words through their previous health care studies or through their jobs, but grouping the words together sometimes makes it easier to study the set. Explanations of the words are rarely given in the lists themselves. Rather, the explanations of the words emerge in the vocabulary exercises, dialogues, or class discussions.

Communication Strategy

Mastery of the communication strategies included in this textbook—whether they be a speech act (e.g., agreeing, apologizing, or giving advice), a confirmation or comprehension check, or a non-verbal cue or gesture—is crucial for success in the health care field. Health care workers who do not speak English as a first language need to learn how to avoid or repair a communication breakdown when speaking with clients, colleagues, or supervisors. When teaching each lesson, the instructor must make sure that students understand the meaning behind each strategy before they begin the exercises. Additional phrases that arise during the lesson can be added to the list. Common idiomatic phrases have been added when appropriate.

Pronunciation

The Pronunciation sections, many of which are contextualized, cover the main suprasegmentals (intonation, stress, and rhythm) of English. Some basic sounds (e.g., /ch/, /th/) are also practiced. We avoided use of the IPA and other technical pronunciation content where possible, but in a few cases it was the only way to focus on common problems (like *-ed* vs. *t* or the schwa). The instructor must model the pronunciation of the key phrases for the students to repeat and then allow students to have ample time to practice. The textbook uses visual cues to make pronunciation rules clear. For example, black dots help students visualize the stressed syllables and bold type makes it easier for students to focus on particular sounds. When students are practicing any of the exercises in the text like the dialogues, they should be encouraged to sound as natural as possible. That is, correcting a student's pronunciation should not be limited to the pronunciation sections of the textbook.

Dialogue Review

The Dialogue Review serves as a bridge between the Dialogue and the role plays. At this point, students will be able to review and identify the featured vocabulary items and communication strategies that appeared in the dialogue from the beginning of the section. By comparing their answers with a partner, they are again exposed to the language and have the opportunity to practice.

Role Plays

Role play exercises contain seven scenarios. The role plays may be practiced in pairs or groups of three as noted.

- Students may briefly read all scenarios.
- Students may practice the scenarios while the instructor circulates to decide who will perform which role play for the class.
- Students may be assigned one of the scenarios to develop more thoroughly before performing for the class.

End-of-Unit Discussion

This sharing exercise gives students the opportunity to produce the language features rather than merely practicing them. In addition to being able to give their opinions and exchange ideas on a topic, students can discuss how various issues affect them personally.

Culture Point

The Culture Point is in the form of a story. The characters in the stories are health care workers and clients. After reading the story, students must determine why a misunderstanding has occurred. Although students are very familiar with their own cultures, they may lack the knowledge of how to interact with clients and colleagues who come from different cultural backgrounds. This exercise allows for personal and professional growth. Possible explanations are given on pages 231–32.

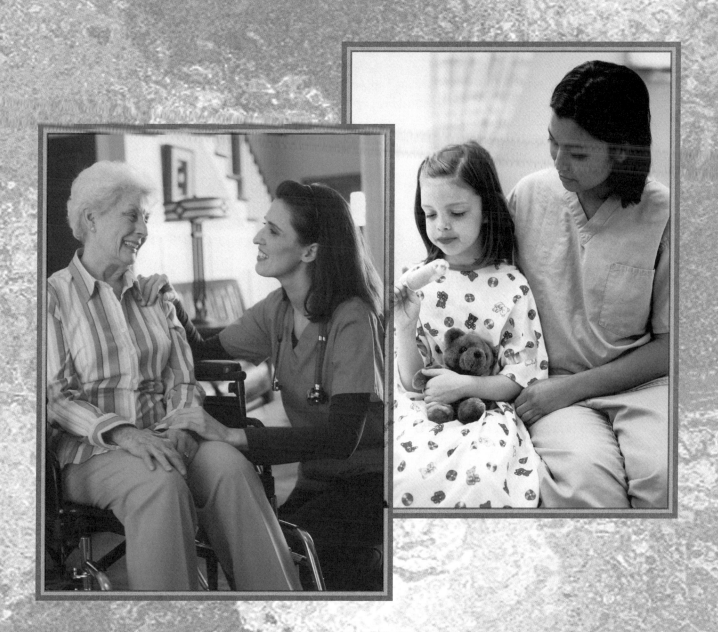

PART 1

Communicating with Clients

UNIT 1: Talking with Clients

Communication between nurses and clients happens all day, every day. At times the communication is formal, such as when a nurse instructs a client how to use a piece of equipment. At other times the topic of communication is informal; for example, the nurse greets the client, they exchange some small talk, and then the nurse moves to the next room

Meeting Clients

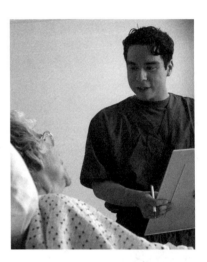

Most people who work in a health care profession are, of course, involved with clients every day. Some clients spend a lot of time in the hospital. In these cases, the nurses and various doctors and specialists will get to know them well. Other clients are only in the hospital a day or two. Still others are in a hospital as outpatients (their surgery or procedure takes place during the day and they go home the same night). Health care workers need to react appropriately to whatever news the client gives.

Listening to the Action

Listening for Language

Listen to the conversations between health care workers and clients. What phrases do the health care workers use to react to the clients' news?

1. _____

2. _____

3. _____

⇅ Dialogue

Practicing the Language

It's been a busy day at Rossmoor Medical Center. The nurse is at the end of her shift, but a new client has been admitted, so she stops by to check on her. Practice the dialogue with a partner.

Nurse: Good morning, Mrs. Chan. My name is Evelyn, and I'll be one of the nurses taking care of you here.

Client: Nice to meet you. You look really young to be a nurse!

Nurse: Really? That's nice to hear. I've been a nurse for three years now.

Client: Well, I guess everyone is young compared to me. I'm just 72 years "young."

Nurse: Good for you! Well, I see that you are here for a hip replacement.

Client: Yes, my orthopedic surgeon will come to see me soon.

Nurse: Are you nervous?

Client: Not really.

Nurse: Will someone from your family be here with you?

Client: Yes . . . I think I hear them now.

Nurse: Great! Well, my shift is over and I need to leave now, but I'll be back tomorrow at 7:00 AM. Good luck with your surgery.

Client: Thanks.

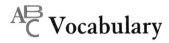 Vocabulary

Medical Specialists

There are many types of health care workers. Clients generally start by seeing a general practitioner, but then they are referred to a specialist. If you work at a hospital or clinic, you will interact with a variety of specialists.

Matching Types of Specialists

Match the type of specialist on the left with the correct area of specialty on the right.

1. allergist _____

2. cardiologist _____

3. dermatologist _____

4. gastroenterologist _____

5. hematologist _____

6. neurologist _____

7. ophthalmologist _____

8. orthopedic surgeon _____

9. otolaryngologist _____

10. pediatrician _____

11. podiatrist _____

12. psychiatrist _____

a. mental or emotional issues

b. heart diseases

c. eye injuries or diseases

d. children's health issues

e. skin diseases

f. allergies

g. foot problems

h. musculoskeletal system issues

i. blood diseases

j. nervous system issues

k. stomach problems

l. ear, nose, and throat problems

Defining More Specialists

Clients may ask you about the area that some specialists work in. In simple language, write what these specialists do. Use a dictionary if you need to. The first one has been done for you as an example.

1. internist: *treats diseases of the structures inside a body* _____

2. anesthesiologist: _____

3. obstetrician/gynecologist: _____

4. pathologist: _____

5. plastic surgeon: _____

6. urologist: _____

⇆ Communication Strategy

Verbal Cues

When you are listening to a client talk and you want to show that you are listening, you can use verbal cues. You also need to show the person talking that you are interested. One way to communicate these messages is with a verbal cue as well as with an emotion, such as being happy, sad, or surprised. There are many phrases to use.

I'm listening.
> Uh-huh.
> Mm-hmm.
> Right.
> Yes.
> Go on.

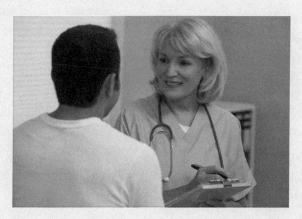

> *Client:* Let me tell you about my pain.
> *Nurse:* Uh-huh.

I'm happy. (That's good news.)
> That's nice.
> Great!
> Congratulations!
> Good for you!

> *Client:* I walked 50 steps yesterday.
> *Nurse:* Congratulations!

I'm sad. (That's bad news.)
> That's too bad.
> Oh, no!
> That's terrible/awful.
> I'm sorry to hear that.

> *Client:* My children won't be able to visit me before the operation.
> *Nurse:* Oh, no.

I'm surprised.
> Really?
> You're kidding!
> Wow!

> *Client:* All 10 of my children were born in this hospital.
> *Nurse:* You're kidding! Wow!

Dialogue Completion

Write an appropriate verbal cue for these statements. The first one has been done for you as an example.

1. Well, this is how it started. Last week. . . .

   Uh-huh.

2. I need to get better. Next month I'm getting married.

   _____

3. I lost my hospital I.D. card.

   _____

4. I have a story about what happened last night.

   _____

5. You look like a movie star!

   _____

6. I think my sister is very sick.

   _____

7. I'm so happy. I don't feel any pain in my shoulder.

   _____

8. I'm the mayor, you know.

   _____

Dialogue Practice

Read and practice the dialogues with a partner.

1. *Nurse's Aide:*   (sees client eating) Did you listen to what the doctor said?
   Client: About what?
   Nurse's Aide: You are not supposed to eat candy bars and things like that.
   Client: Really?
   Nurse's Aide: Yes, really. You need to give those back to your family.
   Client: That's too bad. They are so good!

2. *Client:*   Did you hear my news?
   Nurse: No. What is it?
   Client: My cancer is gone! I'm going to be discharged!
   Nurse: Wow! That's nice.
   Client: Can you come to a party my family is having on Saturday for me?
   Nurse: Sure . . . No, wait. I have to work at that time.
   Client: Oh, I'm sorry to hear that.

Discussion

Work with a small group. Take turns choosing a topic from the list and talking about it for as long as you can. Practice giving verbal cues when your classmates are talking.

1. your favorite food

2. an ideal place to live

3. a difficult subject in school

4. your favorite hobby

5. your favorite movie

⇆ Communication Strategy

Self-Introductions

In the health care field, you meet people every day. Most of the time you are not introduced by someone else. You need to use a self-introduction. After greeting someone, it is important to give your name and explain why you are there.

Nurse: Good morning, Mr. Reynolds. My name's Sunny, and I'm going to be your nurse today.

Client: Nice to meet you. Please call me Sam.

After someone greets you and introduces her/himself to you, it is important to respond (answer) appropriately. Here are some common responses to introductions.

Formal

I'm very pleased/happy/glad to meet you.

It's very nice to meet you.

It's a pleasure to meet you.

It's my pleasure to meet you.

Hello.

Informal

Pleased/Happy/Glad to meet you.

Nice to meet you.

My pleasure.

Hi.

Doctor: Hello. I'm Dr. Robbins, and I'll be examining you today.

Client: Hello, Doctor. I'm very pleased to meet you. You come highly recommended by my friends.

Doctor: That's nice to hear. It's a pleasure to meet you too, Sarah.

Dialogue Completion

Complete the dialogues with appropriate phrases. Use your own names.

1. *Supervisor:* I'm _____. I'll be your supervisor.
   (name)

   New nurse: _____ _____ _____

   Supervisor: _____, too.

2. *Nurse:* Hello, _____. I'm your nurse on this shift. My name is _____.
   (name)   (name)

   Client: _____.

   Nurse: _____.

3. *Nurse's Aide 1:* Hi. I'm _____. I'm one of the nurse's aides here. You must be new?
   (name)

   Nurse's Aide 2: Yes, it's my first day. I'm _____.
   (name)

   Nurse's Aide 1: _____.

   Nurse's Aide 2: _____.

4. *Client:* Good morning. Are you the doctor?

   Nurse: No, I'm your nurse. My name is _____. How are you today?
   (name)

   Client: A little tired. My name is _____, by the way.
   (name)

   Nurse: I'm very happy to meet you, _____.
   (name)

   Client: _____.

Pronunciation: Intonation in Yes-No Questions

A question that can be answered with *yes* or *no* is called a yes-no question. These questions normally begin with a form of the *be* verb, *to do*, *to have*, or a modal (*Can*, *Will*, *Should*, etc.). Listen to your instructor read the yes-no questions. Does the intonation (the "pitch" of the voice) go up (↗) or down (↘)?

1. Is it raining?
2. Wasn't he discharged on Tuesday?
3. Should I include that in her chart?
4. Will you have dinner with me?
5. Does she have plans to become an RN?

<u>Rule</u>: In American English, yes-no questions usually end in rising intonation (↗).

Rising Intonation

Ask the yes-no questions using rising intonation. Take turns asking and answering.

1. Are you busy today?

2. Does your family send you email?

3. Did you study English before you moved to the U.S.?

4. Can you speak a third language?

5. Is anyone in your family a nurse?

6. Will you come to class tomorrow?

7. Would you like to learn about muscle diseases?

8. Have there been any surprises for you in the health care field?

9. Do you know how to provide wound care?

10. Were you nervous on your first day in the hospital?

Writing Questions

Write four yes-no questions, and then ask them to a partner.

1. Do you _____?

2. Are you _____?

3. Can you _____?

4. Will you _____?

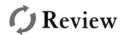 # Review

Dialogue Review

Review the dialogue on page 3. As you read, follow the directions. Then compare your marks with a partner.

- Underline the **Medical Specialist** term.
- Circle the **Verbal Cues.**
- Box the **Self-Introduction** and responses.

Role Plays: Meeting Clients

Work with a partner. Read each situation, and develop dialogues to perform for the class.

1. A specialist introduces himself/herself to a new client in a hospital bed.

2. A nurse listens to a new client's good news and then reacts.

3. An elderly client starts to tell a nurse a long story about the past. The nurse has time to listen and gives verbal cues.

4. A nursing student introduces himself/herself to a client.

5. A client tells a nurse about a lot of new foot pain and asks the nurse what kind of specialist takes care of feet.

6. A nurse introduces himself/herself to a new client and then asks the client two or three yes-no questions.

7. A client tells a nurse's aide about having a lot of bad luck recently and gives examples. The nurse's aide reacts.

Interacting with Clients

Some clients say that hospitals can be interesting places for two or three days, but that after that it's boring to have to stay in a hospital room. Health care workers' interactions with clients (e.g., using small talk and follow-up questions) may make the days a little more interesting.

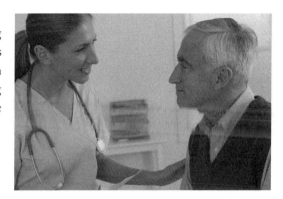

Listening to the Action

Listening for Language

Track 2 3

Listen to the conversations between health care workers and clients. What follow-up questions do the health care workers ask?

1. _____

2. _____

3. _____

Dialogue

Practicing the Language

A nurse is helping a client fill out a form. While she does this, they have a conversation. Practice the dialogue with a partner.

Nurse: Hello, Mr. Dross. I'm here to help you fill out this form for your health insurance company.

Client: Hi. Thanks. My printing's not so good these days.

Nurse: O.K. What is your middle initial?

Client: "X." My middle name is Xavier.

Nurse: Well, that's an interesting name. Now, what's your address, and zip code?

Client: 1320 Elmwood Street. That's in Riverside. The zip code is 92505.

Nurse: All right. What's your date of birth?

Client: June 1st, 1947.

Nurse: Oh, my father was born on June 1st, too. It's a small world! O.K. Now they need to know what medications you're taking. We can get that from your chart. How about substance use? I know that you smoke. How often do you smoke?

Client: I can't smoke in here. In the real world, I smoke about a pack a week—not much.

Nurse: O.K., well, we can fill out the rest of the form based on your chart. We'll submit the form as soon as possible.

Client: Thanks.

Vocabulary

Filling Out Forms

It's part of life to have to fill out forms. People who need medical attention must fill out forms with their personal information and health history. Health professionals must sometimes help them with the forms or even fill out the forms for them.

A Note about Names

In the United States, first names and middle names are chosen at birth by parents. Last names are usually the same as the father's last name. When a woman marries she usually replaces her own last name with that of her husband. Some women in the United States choose to keep their own last name or just add their husband's name after a hyphen, for example: *Mary Deeds-Anderson*.

Recognizing Information on Forms

Categorize each item by the type of information it is. Compare your answers with a partner.

apartment or house number	first name	signature
business (work) phone number	gender (sex)	social security number (S.S.N.)
cell (mobile) phone number	home phone number	state
city	last name (family name)	street
current medications	medical conditions	substance use
date of birth (D.O.B.)	middle initial	zip code
email address	occupation	

Name Information	Address Information	Contact Information	Personal Information	Medical History Information
	apartment or house number			

Filling Out a Form

Write your information in the form.

PERSONAL INFORMATION:

Name: _____ ☐ MALE   ☐ FEMALE
            First   Middle   Last

Address: _____ Apt/Suite: _____

City: _____ State: _____ Zip Code: _____

Home Phone: (_____) _____ - _____ Work Phone: (_____) _____ - _____ EXT. _____

Date of birth: ____/____/_____ AGE: _____

IN CASE OF EMERGENCY, CONTACT: _____ Phone: _____

EMPLOYMENT STATUS:

☐ Full Time   ☐ Part Time   ☐ Retired   ☐ Student   ☐ None

Employer: _____

Address: _____ Suite: _____

City: _____ State: _____ Zip Code: _____

MEDICAL DOCTOR INFORMATION:

Referring Dr: _____ Phone: (_____) _____ - _____

Address: _____ Suite: _____

City: _____ State: _____ Zip Code: _____

Family Dr: _____ Phone (_____) _____ - _____

PLEASE STATE BRIEFLY THE NATURE OF YOUR PROBLEM: _____
_____

LIST MEDICATIONS YOU ARE TAKING: _____
_____

PLEASE LIST OPERATIONS YOU HAVE HAD: _____
_____

PLEASE NAME ANY MEDICATIONS YOU ARE ALLERGIC TO OR HAVE BEEN ADVISED NOT
TO TAKE: _____

Please check any of the following you have had or now have:

☐ Heart Disease   ☐ Cancer   ☐ Emphysema / COPD   ☐ Ringing in ears
☐ Glaucoma   ☐ Back Problems   ☐ Infection / Wounds ☐ Diabetes
☐ Stroke   ☐ Multiple Sclerosis ☐ Tuberculosis   ☐ Circulation
☐ Nausea   ☐ Blood Disorders   ☐ Arthritis   Problems
☐ Artificial Joints ☐ Pacemaker   ☐ Breathing Problems ☐ Epilepsy /
☐ Ulcer Disease   ☐ Asthma   ☐ High Blood Pressure   Convulsions
☐ Depression   ☐ Neck Problems   ☐ Parkinson's Disease

Matching Information

Match the information items on the left with the category on the right.

1. González _____   a. city

2. 6/11/1989 _____   b. zip code

3. 1111 Broadway _____   c. state

4. Long Beach _____   d. last name

5. California _____   e. date of birth (DOB)

6. Rodrigo _____   f. telephone number

7. 90806 _____   g. signature

8. (562) 888-4999 _____   h. address

9. *Rodrigo González* _____   i. first name

⇆ Communication Strategy

Non-Verbal Communication (Facial Expressions)

When talking to a client, health care workers should be conscious of their facial expressions, including their eye contact. Facial expressions contribute to the meaning of what is said.

Emotions from Facial Expressions
disapproval/anger/disgust
disinterest
fear
happiness
interest
pain
sadness
surprise/shock

Eye Contact
avoided
direct
inconsistent
indirect
prolonged

Facial Expressions

Write an appropriate emotion that matches each of these verbal expressions. The first one has been done for you as an example.

1. _____*happiness*_____ "I love you."

2. _____ "Ouch. That hurts!"

3. _____ "That's great!"

4. _____ "Will I die?"

5. _____ "What?!"

6. _____ "I don't care."

Charades

Work in a small group. Take turns choosing one of the emotions in the box on page 14 to act out. You may not talk. The other group members will guess the emotion. Add other emotions that you can think of.

Eye Contact

Which of the types of eye contact from page 14 are being described?

1. _____ A client does not look into the eyes of the nurse. The client looks down at the floor when the nurse is speaking.

2. _____ A doctor looks at the client's eyes when giving the diagnosis.

3. _____ A client's husband looks into her eyes for a long time and lovingly strokes her hair.

4. _____ A nurse looks at a client's eyes, looks away for a second, and then looks at the client's eyes again.

⇆ Communication Strategy

Greetings

A greeting is a friendly way to begin a conversation. In the health care field, it is normal for health care professionals to greet colleagues and clients the first time they see them at the beginning of a shift

Formal	Informal
Good day.	Hey!
Greetings!	Hi!
Good morning/afternoon/evening.	How's it going?
Hello.	What's up?

Nurse 1:   Hi, Abby. How's it going?

Nurse 2:   Hey, Faith. We have a busy day ahead of us!

Greetings

Identify whether each greeting is formal or informal. Circle the answer. Then write a response for each greeting.

1. Hi, Ivan. I heard you got a promotion last week.   formal / informal

   _____.

2. Good morning, Mrs. Fultz. Did you sleep well?   formal / informal

   _____.

3. Hello, Dr. Milton. How are you today?   formal / informal

   _____.

4. How's it going, José? What's new?   formal / informal

   _____.

⇆ Communication Strategy

Small Talk and Follow-Up Questions

Natural conversations have a flow. They start with a topic and expand (get longer and more interesting). One way to expand a conversation is with more questions. Follow-up questions are the second, third, and other questions that you ask about one topic. It is good to ask follow-up questions during small talk with clients, during discussions in a class, or when you are getting to know someone better.

You can use yes-no questions or you can use general information questions using *Who, What, When, Where, Why,* or *How (Wh-* questions).

Yes-No Questions

"My son was here yesterday to visit me."

Is he your only child?

Are you happy that he came?

Do you like to have visitors?

Does he have children?

Can you tell me about him?

Will he come again?

Wh- **Questions**

"I am from Manila."

Who else from your family is in the United States?

What is the weather like in Manila?

When did you leave there?

Where is Manila?

Why did you want to leave Manila?

How is life different in the Philippines?

Sentence Completion

Complete the sentences with an appropriate question word.

1. _____ they your son's children or your daughter's children?

2. _____ she want to move here to be with you?

3. _____ you mind telling me the story?

4. _____ kind of food does he like?

5. _____ did your daughter move away?

Dialogue Completion

Read the dialogues, and add two follow-up questions.

1. A: Are you from a big city?

   B: No, I'm not.

   _____

   _____

2. A: What are you going to do after you're discharged?

   B: I'm going to relax.

   _____

   _____

3. A: What happened?

   B: I lost my glasses!

   _____

   _____

Dialogue Practice

Compare your answers with a partner. Then practice each of your dialogues, asking and answering questions.

Following Up

Ask your partner these questions. Listen to the answer. Then ask a follow-up question, listen to the answer, and ask another follow-up question.

Partner A	Partner B
1. How many people are in your family?	1. Where is your favorite place to travel?
2. Where have you traveled?	2. How long have you been in the United States?
3. Can you play any sports?	3. What kind of music do you like?
4. What is your favorite food?	4. Do you like spicy food?

Pronunciation: Intonation in *Wh-* Questions

Wh- questions require longer answers. They always start with a question word. *Wh-* questions can be affirmative or negative. Listen to your instructor read the *wh-* questions. Does the intonation (the "pitch" of the voice) go up (↗) or down (↘)?

1. Where was the accident?

2. When can you sign the form?

3. Which book do you want your wife to bring from home?

4. Why was the cafeteria empty this evening?

5. Who came to visit?

Rule: In American English, *wh-* questions usually end in falling intonation (↘).

Falling Intonation

Ask the *wh-* questions using falling intonation. Take turns asking and answering.

1. How did you sleep last night?

2. Who taught you how to give an injection?

3. When did you have your surgery?

4. Why are you always so happy?

5. How many nurses are going to take care of me today?

6. Which area of the hospital is the most interesting?

7. What time is it?

8. Where is a good place to put this photo of my family?

9. Whose work station is the farthest?

10. When is dinner time?

Writing Questions

Write four *wh-* questions, and then ask them to a partner.

1. What _____ ?

2. When _____ ?

3. Where _____ ?

4. Who _____ ?

Small Talk

Read the yes-no question, answer *yes,* and then write a follow-up *wh-* question with a partner. The first one has been done for you as an example.

1. Do you watch TV? (↗) ___What's your favorite show? (↘)_____

2. Does he greet you every morning? (↗) _____ ?

3. Is your son married? (↗) _____ ?

4. Do you have a middle initial? (↗) _____ ?

5. Should we bring more bandages? (↗) _____ ?

6. Is she addicted to any substance? (↗) _____ ?

7. Can you name the specialty you are most interested in right now? (↗) _____ ?

8. Do you want juice with your meal? (↗) _____ ?

9. Have you met your specialist? (↗) _____ ?

⟳ Review

Dialogue Review

Review the dialogue on page 11. As you read, follow the directions. Then compare your marks with a partner.

- Underline the **Filling Out Forms** terms.
- Circle the **Small Talk Comments**.
- Box the **Greetings.**

Role Plays: Interacting with Clients

Work with a partner. Read each situation, and develop dialogues to perform for the class.

1. A nursing assistant greets the supervisor at the beginning of a shift and makes small talk.

2. A client doesn't talk much, but shows facial expressions of disinterest, sadness, fear, and pain while a nurse is talking.

3. An allergist greets a client, introduces him/herself, and asks questions and follow-up questions about the client's allergies.

4. A nurse learns that one client is a professional singer. The nurse makes small talk and asks follow-up questions.

5. One nurse greets another nurse who has just returned from a two-week vacation.

6. A nurse is helping a client fill out a form. The nurse asks about the client's current medications, substance use, and medical conditions.

7. A client avoids eye contact and does not use small talk with a nurse's aide who is trying to fill out a form.

End-of-Unit Discussion

Sharing

Discuss the questions with a small group.

1. Which are easier for you—verbal cues (in response to something you hear) or non-verbal cues?

2. If you are making small talk with someone, what are your favorite topics?

3. What are some challenges you might have when you help clients fill out forms?

4. Do you think it is necessary to introduce yourself to each client? What if you are only going to be in a client's room for a short time?

Culture Point: Smiling

Read this story. Discuss it in small groups and as a class.

Nurse Gabrielle was teaching a client how to give himself injections of Vitamin B12. The client, Mr. Vong, was not doing a very good job. He seemed to be too nervous to learn. Gabrielle saw that he was smiling. She thought that he was not concentrating enough and didn't really want to learn. Their conversation follows.

Gabrielle: Mr. Vong. You need to be serious. It's very important for you to learn how to give yourself these injections.

Mr. Vong: I'm sorry, Ma'am (smiling).

Gabrielle: Maybe you need to try it with a different nurse.

Why was Gabrielle so frustrated with Mr. Vong?

UNIT 2: Managing Different Types of Clients

In addition to helping clients who are 18 to 65 years old (adults), health care workers must frequently help the elderly (*geriatric* clients) and young people (*pediatric* clients). The type of communication used with the different groups must be age-appropriate.

Working with the Elderly

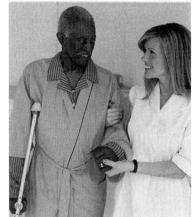

It may be challenging to work with elderly clients. Many elderly people may not hear well, so health care workers must speak slowly and clearly and make sure that the client is listening and comprehending (understanding). It is also important to learn how to say "no" politely when speaking to the elderly.

Listening to the Action Track 4

Listening for Language

Listen to the conversations. What phrases do the health care workers use to make sure the other person is listening?

1. _____

2. _____

3. _____

⇅ Dialogue

Practicing the Language

A 75-year-old man has been admitted to the hospital because he has been fainting recently. His wife called 9-1-1 when he fainted in the kitchen. The paramedics decided that he should go to the hospital. He is talking with a certified nursing assistant (CNA). Practice the dialogue with a partner.

Nursing Assistant: Good morning, Mr. Senich. How are you today?

Client: Eh?

Nursing Assistant: I said, "Good morning. How are you?"

Client: Oh, fine, fine. I'm the picture of health.

Nursing Assistant: I'm Greta Levis. I'm going to be assisting you today. Right now I need to take your blood pressure.

Client: Humph!

Nursing Assistant: I need to you relax as I do this. Is that clear?

Client: Look, I'm not sick. I need to get out of here. My wife needs me at home.

Nursing Assistant: I'm afraid that's not possible, Mr. Senich. The paramedics brought you here last night because of your fainting. The doctors need to watch you as they wait for your test results. Dr. Seefelt will be here soon to talk with you.

Client: Oh, all right. If you say so.

🄰🄱🄲 Vocabulary

Terms of Address

English has only a few terms of address, words used to refer to people. Your native language might have more. It is important to use the correct term. If you use the wrong term, the clients or family members may not understand that you are talking to them. Here are some terms to use with a person's last name.

- Dr. (for men or women who are medical doctors or who have a Ph.D.)
- Nurse (for men or women who have a nursing degree)
- Mr. (for men)
- Ms. (for women)
- Mrs. (for married women who ask you to call them Mrs.)

Note: For children and young people, no address term and no last name is needed.

Other address terms are used without a person's last name.

- Sir (for men)
- Ma'am (for older women)
- Miss (for younger women)
- Officer
- Chaplain/Father/Reverend/Pastor

Note: *Doctor* and *Nurse* may also be used without a last name.

Note: If clients or family members want to change the formality of the relationship, they will ask you to use their first name.

Using Terms of Address

Read the situations. Work with a partner to write short dialogues with appropriate terms of address based on how formal or informal the relationship is. Present one to the class. The first one has been done as an example.

1. A nurse meets a client.

   Nurse: Good morning, Mrs. Walker. My name is Donna, and I'm going to be your nurse today.

   Client: Oh, please call me Helen.

   Nurse: O.K., Helen. It's nice to meet you.

   Client: It's nice to meet you too.

2. A doctor meets a client.

3. A nurse meets the mother of a client.

4. The hospital chaplain meets a new nurse's aide.

5. A nurse meets a physical therapist.

6. The head of nurses meets the new hospital staff psychiatrist.

Choosing the Appropriate Terms of Address

Read the situations. Then decide which address term, if any, you would use to get the attention of each person. The first one has been done as an example.

1. You see an elderly man drop his wallet. _Excuse me, Sir. You dropped your wallet._

2. You see a little girl drop her doll. _____

3. You see a nurse drop his pen. _____

4. You see the president of the medical staff forget his paper. _____

5. You see a family member you have met go the wrong direction. _____

6. You see a woman exit the wrong door. _____

7. You see a police officer lose her notepad. _____

8. You see a young boy forget his jacket. _____

9. You see a doctor you don't know leave her cell phone on the desk. _____

⇆ Communication Strategy

Comprehension Checks

Geriatric clients may not always focus on what you are saying. When you need to know that someone is listening to you, you can use extra phrases to check this. These phrases are called **comprehension checks.** There are many formal and informal phrases to use.

Formal

Excuse me. Have you been listening to me?

I am sorry. I was wondering if you heard what I just said/asked.

Pardon me. Did you understand me just then?

Less Formal

Did you hear what I just said/asked?

Can you hear me?

Informal

Did you catch that?

Did you get that?

Got that?

Right?

Dialogue Practice

Read and practice these dialogues with a partner.

1. *Nurse:*   Mr. Chávez, we need to know which juice you'd like for breakfast.

   Client: Ummm . . . juice?

   Nurse: Did you hear what I just asked?

   Client: Uh . . . what? Oh, yeah. O.K. Apple.

   Nurse: Thank you.

2. *Nursing Assistant 1:* Remember that Mr. Fisher in 212-B needs his dentures cleaned.

   Nursing Assistant 2: La la la. [singing]

   Nursing Assistant 1: Got that?

   Nursing Assistant 2: Huh?

   Nursing Assistant 1: Mr. Fisher, 212-B, needs his dentures cleaned.

   Nursing Assistant 2: Oh, yes. Right away.

Writing Dialogues

Write your own dialogues with partner. Then read them for the class. The first one has been started.

1. *Nurse:* _____.

   Client: Ummm . . .

   Nurse: _____ . _____

   _____

   Client: Uh . . . what? Oh, yeah. O.K. _____.

   Nurse: I hope you understand. Thank you.

2. *A:* _____

   B: _____

   A: _____

   B: _____

Discussion

Take turns talking about the topics with a partner. Use comprehension checks to make sure your partner is listening.

1. Your best experience with a client (or as a client)

2. Your worst experience with a client (or as a client)

3. Your favorite place in a medical facility

4. Your least favorite place in a medical facility

⇆ Communication Strategy

Refusals

Sometimes it's necessary to say no when a person makes a request or tries to do something that is not allowed. It might be possible to just say no, but most of the time you need to use a longer phrase. It is also a good idea to explain why the answer is no.

Formal

Sorry. That's impossible.
I'm afraid that's not possible.
That's out of the question.
You cannot/must not do that.

Less Formal

No, that's not a good idea.

Informal

Absolutely not.
No.
No way.
Not a chance.
Thumbs down.

Dialogue Practice

Read and practice the dialogues with a partner.

1. *Doctor:*   Are you going to work a double shift today?

   Nurse: Sorry. That's impossible today.

2. *Nurse 1:*   You're tired. Let me take your second shift today.

   Nurse 2:   No way! You're just as tired as I am.

3. *Client:*   Can you get me some coffee, please?

   Nurse: No, that's not a good idea with your condition.

Dialogue Completion

Complete the dialogues with a refusal. Add another sentence to explain the answer.

1. *Client:*   It's my birthday today. Can I have a party here?

   You: _____.

2. *Doctor:*   I would like to talk to this client's family immediately.

   You: _____.

3. *Family Member:*   Is it O.K. if I sleep in the waiting room tonight?

   You: _____.

Pronunciation: Stress in Names

Most first names in English have two or three syllables. It is important to pronounce names correctly. Listen to your instructor read the names. The dot (•) marks the stress.

• Wayne Dickerson	• Ms. Hahn	• Mr. Kennedy
• Dr. Doughton	• Dr. Grey	• Dr. Salazar
• Nurse Brenner	• Nurse Skokut	• Nurse Nakane

Rule: The first syllable of the last name usually carries the stress. Many last names follow the same pattern. The last name carries more stress than the first name. When using a title and last name, the pattern is the same.

Practicing Name Stress

Mark the stress on these names, and then practice the pronunciation with a partner. Use the phrase *I'd like you to meet* before each name.

1. Mrs. Berry
2. Nurse Zhang
3. Dr. Wistrom
4. Margaret Hoolihan

5. Mr. Blake
6. Nurse Ratchett
7. Dr. Mitchell
8. Angela Barton

9. Ms. Koupai
10. Nurse Woo
11. Dr. Luck
12. Marcus Bennett

Using Names in Conversation

Answer the questions in a small group.

1. Who was the first person you saw today (in class or at work)?

2. Who is your favorite singer or actor?

3. Who is the president of the United States? Who is the leader of your native country?

4. Who is your favorite television nurse or television doctor?

5. How do you introduce yourself to others using your complete name?

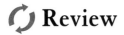 Review

Dialogue Review

Review the dialogue on page 24. As you read, follow the directions. Then compare your marks with a partner.

- Underline the **Address** terms.
- Circle the **Comprehension Check for Listening.**
- Box the **Refusal.**

Role Plays: Dealing with the Elderly

Work with a partner. Read each situation, and develop dialogues to perform for the class.

1. A hospital worker meets an elderly client who does not want to stay in the hospital.

2. An elderly woman goes to the doctor's office because she is experiencing chest pains. The receptionist does the initial assessment.

3. An elderly woman does not believe that she needs to go to the hospital after falling. She talks to the emergency medical technician.

4. An elderly client who doesn't hear well meets a new nurse. The nurse needs to check the client's vital signs.

5. A nurse's aide takes information from an elderly client. The client doesn't want to give much information.

6. An elderly man with a hearing problem refuses to wear his hearing aids. A nurse tries to tell him that it's time for his physical therapy session.

7. A nurse spends extra time with a client who is lonely. The nurse tries to make the client feel better.

Working with Young People

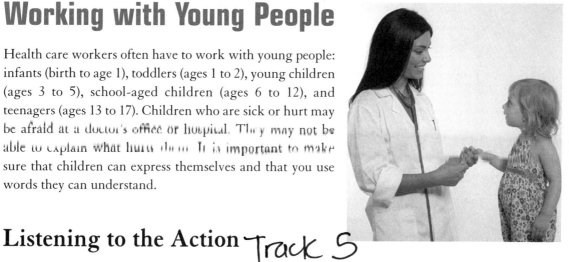

Health care workers often have to work with young people: infants (birth to age 1), toddlers (ages 1 to 2), young children (ages 3 to 5), school-aged children (ages 6 to 12), and teenagers (ages 13 to 17). Children who are sick or hurt may be afraid at a doctor's office or hospital. They may not be able to explain what hurts them. It is important to make sure that children can express themselves and that you use words they can understand.

Listening to the Action Track 5

Listening for Language

Listen to the conversations between health care workers and pediatric clients. What specific age-appropriate words do the health care workers use?

1. _____

2. _____

3. _____

Dialogue

Practicing the Language

Senan is four years old and is in the hospital with several broken bones. His mother is with him when the nurse who comes on shift enters the room. Practice the dialogue in groups of three.

Nurse: Hello, Senan. My name is Ray, and I'm going to be your nurse today.

Good morning, Mrs. Babol. How is he doing today?

Mother: He's in a better mood than yesterday. I brought him his favorite toys.

Nurse: Hey, Senan. That's a cool robot. Does it beat up on the bad guys?

Client: Yeah, and it talks, too.

Nurse: Awesome! Hey, I'm going to listen to your heart with this round metal thing. Do you want to listen to you robot's heart first?

Client: Robots don't have hearts!

Nurse: Oh, right, sorry. Well, can you tell me where you have an owie today?

Client: This part [points to shoulder] and this part [points to thigh] and this part and this part and this part. [points all over his body and begins to laugh]

Nurse: Oh! Did you break all of the bones in your body?

Client: Yeah.

Nurse: I bet there's one bone that didn't break. You didn't break your funny bone! [tickles Senan on the arm]

Client: You're funny!

Nurse: We'll fix up your bones, but you have to promise no more climbing trees. You and Mr. Robot need to stay on the ground.

ABC Vocabulary

Age-Appropriate Words and Phrases

Toddlers and young children may use different words and expressions than adults use when they talk about their bodies or illnesses. It is useful to know which words you might try when talking to a child.

Child-specific vocabulary includes words for pain, injuries, clothing, family members, and other items.

- **Pain:** Ouch! / Ow!
- **Injury:** Owie! / Boo-boo
- **Body Parts:** tummy
- **Family Members:** Mommy, Daddy Mama, Papa
- **Clothing:** jammies / PJs
- **Items:** dolly, Teddy Bear, rubber duckie, blankie

Ask the parents which verbs they use at home for these personal issues.

- toileting (to go potty, pee / pee-pee / #1, poo / poo-poo / #2)
- eating (All done!)
- bathing (Bath time!)

Recognizing Age-Appropriate Words

Write a more formal word for the words that young children sometimes use. Then think of three others you are familiar with.

1. tummy   *stomach*   7. _____   _____

2. PJs   _____   8. _____   _____

3. boo-boo   _____   9. _____   _____

4. Mommy   _____

5. potty   _____

6. blankie   _____

Dialogue Completion

Complete the conversations using the words from the list on page 32.

1. *Pediatric Client:*   Oooooh . . .

   Nurse's Aide: Do you have to go _____?

   Pediatric Client: Uh-huh.

   Nurse's Aide: _____ or _____?

2. *Pediatric Client:*   I like your clothes with all of those yellow duckies.

   Pediatric Nurse: And I like your cute _____ with those little monkeys.

3. *Pediatric Client:*   Waaaaa!

   Nurse's Aide: Look who's here! Your _____ and _____ are here to be with you all day.

⇆ Communication Strategy

Invented Words or Euphemisms

When talking with toddlers or young children, you may have to invent some words because children may not understand the technical term. It's best to use a **euphemism** (a word that is used in place of a word that might be too direct, harsh, or scary).

Euphemisms
  bed on wheels
  picture of your bones
  poke
  sleepy air
  sore
  wake-up room

Matching

Match the technical word in the left column with the euphemism in the right column.

1. anesthesia _____   a. bed on wheels

2. shot _____   b. picture of your bones

3. stretcher_____   c. poke

4. recovery room _____   d. sore

5. pain _____   e. sleepy air

6. x-ray _____   f. wake up room

Inventing Euphemisms

Invent a word or phrase for each technical word or phrase that would be appropriate to use with children. Share your ideas with a small group.

1. stethoscope _____

2. blood pressure cuff _____

3. antiseptic _____

4. privacy screen _____

5. chemotherapy _____

6. CT scan _____

Writing Dialogues

With a partner, write your own dialogue between a nurse and a child. Use euphemisms. Then read it to the class.

⇆ Communication Strategy

Distracting Someone

When talking to children, you might have to change the topic or use a special phrase in order to distract them from their pain or from a procedure.

Hey, let's try this.

Hey, why don't we

Let's count to three. One, two, three.

Look at me.

High five! Now low five!

Just relax.

You're such a big girl/boy.

Dialogue Completion

Complete the dialogues with phrases from the box on page 34. The first one has been done for you as an example.

1. *Pediatric Client:* I don't want a bandage on my head!

   Nurse: Hey, let's try this. We can make Mr. Bear be the patient and you be the

   doctor. You can put the bandage on Mr. Bear and see how he looks

2. *Pediatric client:* I don't like needles. I want my Mommy!

   Nurse: _____

   _____

3. *Pediatric client:* Waaaaa! Owwwww!

   Nurse: _____

   _____

4. *Pediatric client:* Can I go home today?

   Nurse: _____

   _____

Using Language to Distract Children

Write an appropriate phrase to distract a child in each situation. Share your ideas with a small group.

1. A 2-year-old girl who won't go to sleep: _____

2. A 4-year-old boy who is getting an injection: _____

3. A 5-year-old girl who just broke her arm: _____

4. A 6-year old boy who is in pain: _____

Pronunciation: Stress in Adjective-Noun Pairs

It is common to describe a noun in English. Listen to your instructor read the adjective-noun pairs. Which word gets the stress?

1. dirty bathroom   2. delicious food

<u>Rule</u>: In most adjective-noun pairs, the noun has more stress than the adjective.

<u>Note</u>: If the speaker wants to focus on the adjective (e.g., when giving a compliment), then the adjective has more stress than the noun.

Adjective-Noun Pair Stress

Mark the stress on these adjective-noun pairs, and then practice the pronunciation with a partner. Use the phrase *That looks like* before each phrase.

1. a nice doll	5. a happy child	9. cold milk
2. a new shirt	6. a good book	10. bad weather
3. a fun game	7. a tired patient	11. your big brother
4. a worried parent	8. an upset tummy	12. blue slime

Stressing the Adjectives

Now read the 12 adjective-noun pairs, but put the stress on the adjective. Work with a partner.

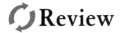# Review

Dialogue Review

Review the dialogue on pages 31–32. As you read, follow the directions. Then compare your marks with a partner.

- Underline the **Child-Specific terms.**
- Circle the **Euphemisms.**
- Box the **Phrases Used to Distract Children.**

Role Plays: Dealing with Young People

Work with a partner. Read each situation, and develop a dialogue to perform for the class.

1. A nurse tries to calm down a six-year-old client whose parents have just left the hospital.

2. A mother brings her little boy to the doctor's office. She says that he's been complaining about pains in his legs. The doctor tries to determine what's wrong.

3. A young cancer client will go into the hospital for her first chemotherapy treatment. Her mother tries to prepare her for what will happen.

4. A little girl falls on the playground and needs stitches in her chin. A nurse keeps her distracted while the doctor is working on the wound.

5. A three-year-old girl is afraid to go into surgery. A nurse uses euphemisms to describe what is going to happen.

6. A nurse assistant asks a young client to talk about his toys.

7. A nurse distracts a little girl as she gets an injection.

End-of-Unit Discussion

Sharing

Discuss the questions with a small group.

1. Do you think elderly clients are usually easier or more difficult to work with compared to other clients? Why?

2. Do you mind if a geriatric client calls you *Sweetie* or *Dear?* If you mind, how would you ask them to stop?

3. Which types of clients seem to be most nervous about being in the hospital?

4. What are the advantages and disadvantages of working in a pediatrics ward?

Culture Point: Caring for Children

Read this story. Discuss in small groups and as a class.

An infant girl was going to be discharged from the hospital. While the mother was filling out paperwork at the nurses' station, two nurses in the child's room started to explain to the father how the parents needed to provide child care when they returned home. "Please don't tell me anything," the father said, and he left the room. The nurses were surprised. When the mother came back to the room, she explained why her husband had left.

Why did the father leave?

UNIT 3: Talking with Family Members

Most people who are sick or injured arrive at the hospital with relatives (family members) or friends. Some clients who are admitted to the hospital can have daily visitors. Health care workers need to clearly communicate the client's condition and explain to family members what is happening.

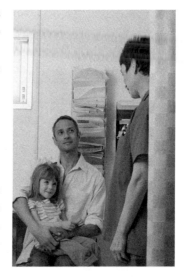

Reporting to Families

When a client enters the Emergency Department, family members are usually very anxious and worried. A health care worker must use simple language to describe the client's condition and explain what is happening. It is also important to learn how the family member is related to the client.

Listening to the Action

Listening for Language

Listen to the conversations between health care workers and family members. Which family members are the health care workers talking to?

1. _____

2. _____

3. _____

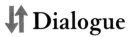 Dialogue

Practicing the Language

Many family members of a burn victim are gathering in the waiting room of Harbor Hospital's Emergency Department. Practice the dialogue in groups of three.

Nurse: May I have your attention, everyone. I know that you are all here for Billy Blair. Can we get one of you to be the representative of the family?

Grandfather: Barbie—you talk to her. She's Billy's wife. [to the nurse]

Wife: I . . . can't. [sobs uncontrollably]

Grandfather: O.K. I'll talk to you. I'm his grandfather. His parents aren't here yet.

                [The nurse and the grandfather move to the hallway outside the trauma rooms.]

Grandfather: Can you tell me Billy's condition?

Nurse: I'm sorry. I can't. It'll be just a little while longer until the doctors let us know.

Grandfather: Well, what do you know right now? I gotta tell the others something.

Nurse: What I know is that the doctors needed to do an emergency tracheotomy.

Grandfather: What does that mean?

Nurse: In simple terms, it means that they had to cut a hole in Billy's neck in order for him to breathe. You'll have to excuse me now. Please go back with the others. I'll keep you posted.

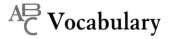 Vocabulary

Words for Family

Family members or relatives often identify themselves when they speak with doctors or nurses at a medical center. They will sometimes say how they are related to the client, such as, *I'm his brother* or *We're his parents.* It may not be necessary to ask the relative his or her name; just knowing the relationship may be enough.

There are many types of family members, both immediate and extended.

- **Grandparents:** grandmother (grandma), grandfather (grandpa)
- **Parents:** mother (mom), father (dad)
- **Spouse:** wife, husband
- **Children:** daughter, son
- **Siblings:** sister, brother, twin
- **Extended Family:** aunt, uncle, niece, nephew, cousin
- **Family by Marriage:** mother-in-law, father-in-law, sister-in-law, brother-in-law, daughter-in-law, son-in-law
- **Other Family:** stepmother, stepfather, stepdaughter, stepson, stepsister, stepbrother, next-of-kin

Using Vocabulary about Family

Fill in the blanks with the appropriate family member vocabulary word.

1. Your father's wife is your _____.

2. A son of your uncle is your _____.

3. Your husband's sister is your _____.

4. A female child of your parents is your _____.

5. Your male child is your _____.

6. Your mother's father is your _____.

7. Your son's wife is your _____.

8. You are married to your _____.

Sentence Completion

Write sentences to describe these family members.

1. _____ is your son-in-law.

2. _____ is your grandmother.

3. _____ is your aunt.

4. _____ is your brother.

5. _____ is your father-in-law.

6. _____ is your daughter.

Discussion

Discuss with a partner how many of each family member you have.

1. sisters

2. uncles

3. nephews

4. cousins

⇆ Communication Strategy

Rephrasing Language

Health care workers use medical jargon with each other. **Jargon** refers to the technical words and phrases for a field. With clients and relatives, health care workers need to use **lay terms**. Lay terms refer to the language that adults use and understand (i.e., their everyday language). There are specific phrases that people use when they explain something technical in lay terms or everyday language for someone not in the same field.

Rephrasing Language

In other words, / In everyday words,

In other terms, / In layperson's terms, / In simple terms,

In language that you can understand,

Let me explain it in simpler terms.

Let me clear things up for you.

Let me give it to you straight.

I'll be as simple and straightforward as I can be.

_____ means _____.

Here are some commonly used "everyday" terms health care workers use.

Technical vs. Everyday Terms

1. ambulate   →   walk
2. defecate   →   bowel movement (BM)
3. edema   →   swelling due to trapped fluid
4. tachycardia   →   increased heart rate
5. void   →   urinate

<u>Note</u>: Most medical abbreviations need to be translated for clients.

Dialogue Completion

Complete the dialogues using a phrase from the box on page 42. Then read and practice them with a partner.

1. *Relative:* I speak perfect English, but I really don't understand what's going on around here! Why do all of you use technical language? I just want to know if my son is going to make it!

   Nurse: Calm down, Mrs. Harrison _____ _____, your son does have critical injuries. He's in surgery now. I'll let you know what the doctors say the minute they finish.

2. *Doctor:* Your wound is draining. We'll need to irrigate it and pack it with gauze. [Doctor leaves.]

   Client: Can you translate what she said?

   Nurse: Yes. _____. Pus is coming out of your wound. We'll need to wash it and then put gauze and bandages on it.

3. *Nurse:* You need to ambulate today.

   Client: Huh?

   Nurse: Sorry. *Ambulate* means "_____." You need to _____ today.

Translating into Everyday Terms

Write an explanation in everyday terms for each situation. Use a dictionary if you need to. Share your ideas with a small group.

1. The client has a bowel obstruction and must have an exploratory surgery.

   _____.

2. The oncoming nurse will hang a new I.V. bag.

   _____.

3. A debridement of the client's wounds will be scheduled.

   _____.

4. Doctors will treat the edema, but you'll be admitted to the hospital.

   _____.

⇆ Communication Strategy

Making Excuses

Excuses are usually used when making an apology, when declining an invitation, and when saying good-bye. When dealing with a client's family members, you may need to make an excuse if something they want is not available (e.g., information) or possible (e.g., a "miracle"). You can start an excuse with one of these common phrases.

> I regret that
>
> I wish I could, but
>
> I'm sorry, I can't.
>
> I'd like to help, but
>
> I know that this is very hard/confusing for you, but
>
> You'll have to pardon me now, but
>
> It's too bad, but

Dialogue Completion

Complete the dialogues with an appropriate phrase from the box.

1. *Relative:* But I'm his cousin. I need to see him!

   Nurse: _____ the doctor's orders are that only the
   immediate family may visit him right now.

2. *Relative:* That's my only child! Promise me that she'll be O.K.

   Nurse: _____ the doctors are doing everything they
   can for her.

3. *Relative:* I don't think that her insurance will pay for this. Do you think that the hospital will
   let her stay?

   Nurse: _____ the hospital will eventually demand
   payment from you if you don't have insurance.

Matching

Match the beginning of an excuse in the left column with an appropriate ending of an excuse in the right column. There may be more than one possible answer.

1. You'll have to pardon me, but . . . _____   a. your wife is not responding to the treatment.

2. It's too bad, but . . . _____   b. I can't.

3. We regret that . . . _____   c. that's how hospitals do business

4. I wish I could, but . . . _____   d. he's in a coma. He can't speak.

5. I know that this is very   e. I need to get back to the ED.
   confusing for you, but . . . _____

 # Pronunciation: Verb Endings

When we talk about the things a person does every day, the verbs end with an -s. What letters do the endings sound like? Listen to your instructor read these sentences.

> Every morning Nurse Evans gets up, showers, combs her hair, and brushes her teeth. Then she dresses and drinks a cup of coffee.

<u>Rule:</u> The way that the -s is pronounced depends on the last sound in the word.

Listen and repeat the words after your instructor.

eat → eats	clean → cleans
drink → drinks	listen → listens
shower → showers	smile → smiles
comb → combs	work → works
clean → cleans	learn → learns
visit → visits	care → cares
brush → brushes	bandage → bandages
dress → dresses	watch → watches
apologize → apologizes	finish → finishes
massage → massages	pass → passes
wax → waxes	teach → teaches

<u>Rule:</u> When the last sound in the base form of the verb is a / s /, / z /, / sh /, / ch /, / j /, or / x /, the ending sounds like / iz / and is an extra syllable.

Verb Endings

Write the verbs with an -s ending. Then practice the pronunciation with a partner.

1. see _____   6. walk _____

2. say _____   7. worry _____

3. tell _____   8. make _____

4. explain _____   9. pay _____

5. wait _____   10. help _____

Recognizing Verb Endings

Read the sentences. Circle the verbs that have an /s/ or /iz/ sound ending.

1. Nurse Holloway helps her clients in many ways.

2. She explains what is happening and makes sure that they understand.

3. She listens to their questions and then answers them.

4. She smiles at everyone and laughs at the clients' jokes.

5. Nurse Holloway cares for all her clients very much.

Verb with an Extra Syllable

Write the verbs with an -es ending. Then practice the pronunciation with a partner.

1. relax _____   6. exercise _____

2. stretch _____   7. change _____

3. reach _____   8. assess _____

4. touch _____   9. wash _____

5. push _____   10. advise _____

Recognizing Verbs with an Extra Syllable

Read the sentences. Circle the verbs that have the -es ending.

1. That client exercises in her hospital bed.

2. First, she raises her arms and reaches for the ceiling.

3. Next, she stretches forward and touches her toes.

4. Then she pushes against the bed rails.

5. When she finishes, she relaxes and massages her feet.

Pronunciation Practice

Work with a partner. Decide who does the following tasks—the client or a health care worker? Write C for client and S for staffer on the line. Then use your answer in a complete sentence. The first two have been done for you as examples.

1. __S__ make the bed ⟩ _A hospital staff member makes the beds._

2. __C__ arrange get well cards → _The client arranges her get well cards._

3. _____ take medications → _____

4. _____ watch TV → _____

5. _____ receive visitors → _____

6. _____ measure blood pressure → _____

7. _____ clean the shower → _____

8. _____ file forms → _____

9. _____ eat in bed → _____

10. _____ fold the towels → _____

11. _____ use a bedpan → _____

12. _____ remove the trash → _____

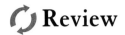 # Review

Dialogue Review

Review the dialogue on page 40. As you read, follow the directions. Then compare your answers with a partner.

- Underline the **Family Members** terms.
- Circle the **Rephrasing Technique**.
- Box the **Making Excuses** phrases.

Role Plays: Reporting to Families

Work with a partner. Read each situation, and develop a dialogue to perform for the class.

1. A client's primary diagnosis is his ineffective airway clearance. A nurse explains this to him in lay terms.

2. A nurse explains to a mother that she may not enter the operating room while her child is in surgery.

3. A client has an extremely rare illness. A doctor tells the client there is a need to consult with experts in another country and there will be a delay in treatment.

4. An accident victim is put on a respirator. A nurse explains to the man's wife what a respirator does.

5. A woman faints in the waiting room when she hears an emergency called. A nurse tells her that it's not for her husband.

6. A nurse calls a pediatric client's family at home to say that the child wants them to bring his homework.

7. A relative starts to make a cell phone call from a client's room, but a nurse stops her and explains hospital policy doesn't allow her to use the phone.

Answering Questions about Visiting Hours

Some clients in the hospital have visitors each day. Getting to know a client's family members can be helpful.

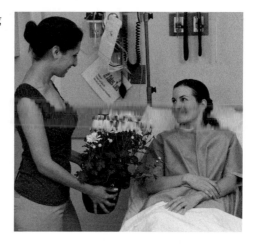

- If the health care worker is teaching a client how to do something, a family member can reinforce the instructions.

- If the client is a non-native speaker of English, a family member can be the interpreter.

Also, talking to a client about family is a nice way to help a client relax or feel better. It is also important to know and provide visiting hour information.

Listening to the Action

 Listening for Language

Listen to conversations between health care workers and family members. What visiting hours do the health care workers provide?

1. _____

2. _____

3. _____

⇅ Dialogue

Practicing the Language

Tuyet Nguyen has just moved to the Sunrise Senior Center, a skilled nursing facility. Her daughter has flown in from Los Angeles to visit, and they are talking in her room. Practice the dialogue in groups of three.

Daughter: Mom, I'm so relieved to see you.

Client: Were you worried? I'm O.K. I'm fine here. Oh! Here's my roommate.

Roommate: Hi. Are you Tuyet's daughter? She told me you were coming. I was just in the hair salon. What do you think? For $20.00?

Daughter: Oh, it's nice to meet you, Sophia, is it? Your hair's beautiful.

Roommate: Well, maybe you should try this style. You're so skinny that some "big hair" might help!

Daughter: Yes, well, maybe. Oh, Mom, let me help you arrange these get well cards.

Client: It's so nice having you here!

Daughter: I'll be here for a few hours today, and I'll come back tonight.

Client: I think that visiting hours end at 8:00 PM.

Daughter: O.K. Hey, is there somewhere I can get something to eat?

Roommate: You are skinny, so you can eat. How much do you weigh?

Client: The vending machines are right down the hall.

Daughter: O.K. I'll be right back. Don't go anywhere—ha ha!

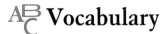 Vocabulary

Emotions

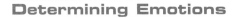

Family members may show a wide range of emotions when they visit a client who is ill or injured. Their emotions may affect the client in a good way (cheerfulness) or a bad way (worry). Health care workers may need to teach relatives how to be good visitors in terms of showing their emotions.

Emotions can be positive or negative.

- **Positive:** cheer, hope, relief
- **Negative:** anger, anxiety, denial, disbelief, exhaustion, fear, frustration, shock, stress, worry
- **Other:** on an emotional roller coaster, surprise

Determining Emotions

Read the situations, and decide which emotions the families may have. There may be more than one appropriate answer. Then compare your answers with a partner.

1. The family learns that the client is being discharged tomorrow. _____

2. The client seems very near death but suddenly sits up to eat some ice cream. _____

3. The family receives a call in the middle of the night to "come to the hospital" because the client's health is deteriorating. _____

4. A doctor tells the family that the client will never walk again. _____

5. The family enters the client's room and finds him on the floor next to the bed. _____

Dialogue Completion

Complete the conversations, and then practice them with a partner.

1. *Nurse:* I know that it's hard to believe, but your father is back in intensive care.

   Relative: We are _____. One day he appears to be fine and the next day he's so sick again.

2. *Nurse:* Mr. Cameron, your son is out of surgery. In the accident, he broke both of his legs and his clavicle.

   Relative: It's all my fault. I'm so _____ with myself. I should have been watching him more carefully.

3. *Nurse:* You have got to take better care of yourself, Mrs. Aquino. Your husband would want you to get some rest.

   Relative: I'm just so _____. I know that you're right. I'll try to get some rest.

⇆ Communication Strategy

Non-Verbal Communication

In addition to using oral English, it is important to know how to use your body when speaking to a client's family members. The non-verbal communication in your culture may be very different from the non-verbal communication of clients and their family members. Non-verbal features can be used in greetings, good-byes, and small talk.

Distance—how much space people leave between speakers
Posture—how people lean, stand, or sit
Handshakes—when and if people shake hands

Comparing Cultures

Complete the chart with what you think is normal for North Americans and what is normal in your culture.

	North American Culture	My Culture
The distance between two people during a conversation		
The posture people use during a conversation		
When and how people shake hands		

The following information is typical for most North Americans.

Distance: In formal conversations, people don't like to be very close to a person when they are speaking. The average distance between two people having a formal conversation should be about one foot. In informal conversations, about half a foot is acceptable.

Posture: In formal conversations, people stand up straight. In informal conversations, a more relaxed posture is acceptable.

Handshakes: In formal situations, people shake hands when being introduced and at the end of a meeting. It is the custom for both men and women to shake hands firmly, but gently. When meeting a client or a relative, handshakes are not necessary.

Practicing Non-Verbal Communication

Line up with half the class members facing the other half. Then follow the directions.

- Have a conversation while standing. First, stand at a distance that is comfortable for you in your culture. Then stand at a distance that is acceptable to North Americans. Demonstrate for the class.
- Have a conversation while standing. First, use formal posture. Then use informal posture. Demonstrate for the class.
- Practice formal introductions in which everyone moves down the line and shakes everyone's hand.

⇆ Communication Strategy

Discussing Visiting Hours

Certain phrases are used by relatives when they come to visit clients. First, the family members need to find the client's room. Then, they may ask about the client's condition. Last, they may need to find another location in the hospital.

Asking about a client or visiting hours

> What time are visiting hours?
> Can I see my mother now?
> I'm trying to locate my mother. Can you help?
> I'm trying to find my mother's room. Can you tell me the room number?
> Can you tell me which room my mother is in? Her name is [ ].

Asking about a client's condition

> How's my mother doing?
> Is she going to be O.K.?
> When can I speak with the doctor?
> My mother is complaining about pain in her legs. Do you know how it is being treated?

Asking about a location

> Can you please tell me where the chapel is?
> Is there a place where I can get something to drink?
> Is there somewhere I can rest for a while?

Dialogue Completion

Complete the dialogues with an appropriate question from the box.

1. *Visitor:* _____?

   Nurse: I'll let the doctor know that you are here.

2. *Visitor:* _____?

   Nurse: I'm sorry, but visiting hours are over at 10:00 PM.

3. *Visitor:* _____?

   Nurse: There's a lounge for families on the 5th floor near the elevators.

4. *Visitor:* _____?

   Nurse: She's in Room 313-A. It's down the hall on the left.

5. *Visitor:* _____?

   Nurse: I'm afraid she's not having a good day today.

⇆ Communication Strategy

Small Talk Topics

Should you make a lot of small talk with clients? It depends. You can if the client isn't busy with visitors. Many clients and their families would like to talk to you.

When using small talk in the United States, some topics are "safe" to talk about but others are "taboo," meaning you should not talk about them. If a topic is not too personal, then it is acceptable to talk about it.

Identifying Acceptable Small Talk Topics

Mark the topics that you think are safe topics to discuss with clients or their family members.

1. food _____

2. hobbies _____

3. holidays _____

4. the hospital _____

5. how much something costs _____

6. local sports teams _____

7. marital status (married, etc.) _____

8. politics _____

9. religion _____

10. someone you both know _____

11. someone's salary _____

12. someone's weight _____

13. weather _____

14. where someone lives _____

Discussion

Discuss these questions in small groups.

1. Did you all check the same topics? Why or why not?

2. Why do you think that some topics are usually safe, while others are not?

3. Are some topics safe only some of the time? Can you give an example from the list?

4. In your country, what topics are usually not safe small talk topics?

Changing the Topic

Start a conversation about a safe topic from the list with a partner. Then ask about a topic that is not safe. Your partner needs to change the conversation back to a safe topic. Reverse roles.

Pronunciation: Basic Sentence Stress

In many languages, sentence stress isn't as strong as it is in English. To sound natural when you speak English, you must practice using proper stress in sentences.

Look at the words. Read and say each word loudly.

nurse   happy   see   patient   visitors

Now, read the sentence containing all of the words. Say the same five words loudly and the other words softly.

The nurse was happy to see the patient have visitors.

Rule: Basic sentence stress in English means some words are stressed and others are not. Nouns, verbs, adjectives, adverbs, question words, and negative words are stressed. Articles, prepositions, pronouns, possessives, conjunctions, and helping verbs are not stressed.

Identifying Stressed Words

Read the sentences, and mark the words that are stressed. Then read them with a partner.

1. Who is the daughter of Mrs. Dankum in Room 204?

2. The young clients were excited to see the famous actor in the hospital.

3. That client is tired but will be happy when her relatives visit.

4. Visiting hours are from 9:00 AM to 9:00 PM.

5. I've worked in this clinic for three years.

Practicing Sentence Stress

Ask your partner the questions using appropriate stress. Write sentences with your partner's answers, and mark the words that have stress. Reverse roles. The first one has been done for you as an example.

1. Question: Where are you from?

   She's from a small town in Pakistan.

2. Question: How many brothers and sisters do you have?

   _____.

3. Question: When did you decide to work in the health care industry?

   _____.

4. Question: Who is your role model?

   _____.

5. Question: Which clinical rotation is your favorite?

   _____.

6. Question: What do you want to do in ten years?

   _____.

Reading for Sentence Stress

Write three sentences about your work or classes today. Mark the stress. Then read one sentence to the class.

   1. _____

   2. _____

   3. _____

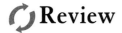 # Review

Dialogue Review

Review the dialogue on pages 49–50. As you read, follow the directions. Then compare your answers with a partner.

- Underline the **Emotions.**
- Circle the **Taboo Topics.**
- Box the **Discussion of Visiting Hours.**

Role Plays: Family Members During Visiting Hours

Work with a partner. Read each situation, and develop dialogues to perform for the class.

1. On the first day a client is admitted to the hospital, her sisters come to look for her. They are having trouble finding her room. They ask a nurse for help.

2. A hospital worker is making small talk with a client's relatives. The worker is trying to avoid taboo topics.

3. The daughter of a client who can't speak English is relaying many complaints and requests to the nurses.

4. Two hospital workers talk to a new client about his family, who will be visiting that afternoon. They ask many questions.

5. A client's children are visiting during dinner time. The client doesn't want to eat the hospital food. The children tell the client that she needs to eat.

6. A husband arrives at the hospital after visiting hours are over. He tries to convince the workers to let him see his wife so that he can kiss her good night.

7. During visiting hours, a client begins to have trouble breathing. The client's relatives run to find a nurse who can help.

End-of-Unit Discussion

Sharing

Discuss the questions with a small group.

1. Which questions from a family member are the hardest to answer? Which type of excuse is the easiest one to give?

2. Why is it important to know who the family members are?

3. What are some ways to deal with the emotions of family members when a client is critically ill?

4. How can you teach relatives how to be good visitors?

Culture Point: Physical Contact

Read this story. Discuss in small groups and as a class.

———

An international student was taken to the hospital with a serious illness. After a week, the student's recovery was going well. Her parents arrived in the United States and went straight to the hospital. As they met the head nurse, they gave her a big hug and kissed her on both cheeks. The nurse was quite surprised and quickly excused herself. She was embarrassed that other hospital staff members saw what happened. The student started to speak excitedly to her parents in their native language.

———

Why was the nurse embarrassed?

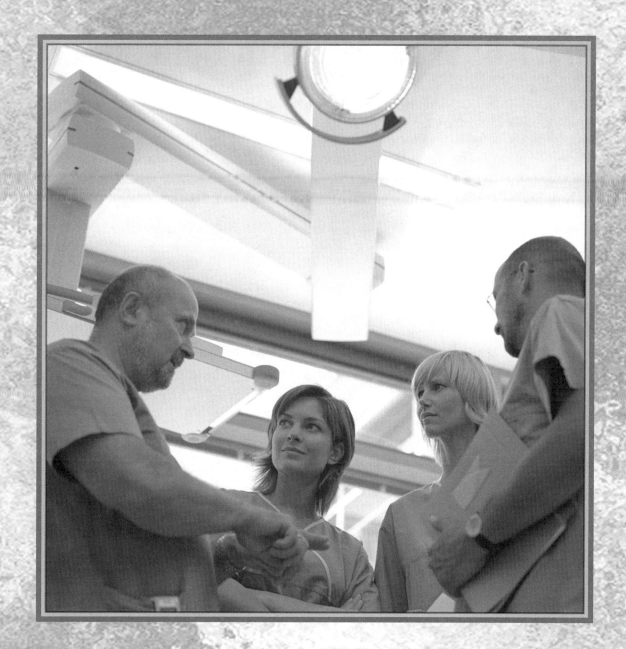

PART 2

Communicating
with Colleagues

UNIT 4: Working with Colleagues

Even though health care workers may work alone sometimes during the day, they will also have to interact with colleagues. Colleagues might exchange pieces of information about a client and make related decisions, help each other with routine tasks, or face an emergency situation together. Communication between colleagues may be formal or informal, but it must always be clear.

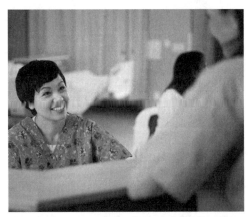

Helping with Tasks

Teamwork is very important in a medical facility. Health care workers must work together closely to provide client care. It's possible that one member of the team has too much to do and needs help from others. In that case, it is possible to request help. After the task is complete, the worker who received help needs to show gratitude.

Listening to the Action

 Listening for Language

Listen to the conversations between colleagues in a health care setting. What specific words do the health care workers use to request help?

1. _____

2. _____

3. _____

⇅ Dialogue

Practicing the Language

On a busy shift, one nurse requests a lot of help from a colleague. Practice the dialogue with a partner.

Nurse 1: Do you need some help?

Nurse 2: Oh, thanks. That would be great. There is just too much going on here today.

Nurse 1: My pleasure. Let me know which clients I can help you with.

Nurse 2: The car accident client in Bed 318-A has asked for more pain meds. Could you possibly get a doctor in to see him?

Nurse 1: Certainly.

Nurse 2: Oh, and the gall bladder operation in 306-A has been complaining about his bed. Do you think you can try to adjust it for him?

Nurse 1: I'll try.

Nurse 2: And the broken leg in 309-B wants someone to fix her TV. Would you mind calling for the technician?

Nurse 1: No problem.

Nurse 2: And, let's see. I just found out that it's Mr. Smith's 70th birthday today. He's in Bed 312-A. I wonder if you could call the kitchen and ask someone to include a candle with his dessert.

Nurse 1: Consider it done.

Nurse 2: And how about teaching me how you keep little Mary in 336 occupied. She's a handful!

Nurse 1: Of course.

Nurse 2: Hmmm. After work, can you go to my house and make dinner for my family? [smiles]

Nurse 1: Sure. [laughing]

ABC Vocabulary

Words Related to Work

There are various words that are used to talk about work. Some of the words have similar meanings. Some of the words are more unique.

- **Nouns:** assignment, duty/responsibility, errand, job, rounds, task, workload
- **Verbs:** to aid/to come to someone's aid, to assist, to help (someone) with, to relieve
- **Idioms:** to lend a hand to, to go to bat for

Dialogue Practice

Read and practice the dialogues with a partner.

1. *Nurse 1:*   Can you help me with the client in Bed 902-A?

   Nurse 2:   Sure. What do you need me to do?

   Nurse 1:   Help him practice using his walker.

2. *Supervisor:* It's time to make your rounds.

   Nurse: Yes, I'm starting right now.

3. *Client:*   Your work seems to be interesting.

   Nurse: Well, some assignments are more interesting than others.

   Client: For example?

   Nurse: Well, working in surgery is very interesting to me.

Sentence Completion

Complete the sentences with an appropriate word from the list on page 61. Change the word as necessary (e.g., make plural). Some sentences have more than one possible answer.

1. Elizabeth had to do many _____ after her shift: go to the bank, take clothes to the dry cleaners, and buy food for dinner.

2. Noreen's _____ increased after two nurses suddenly quit.

3. Pat needs someone to _____ her for 20 minutes while she takes a break.

4. Lillian deserves a promotion. I'm going to _____ her with her supervisor.

5. Emptying the trash seems like a small _____, but it must be done multiple times during the day for hygiene purposes.

Discussion

Write a short answer for each question. Then discuss your answers with a small group.

1. Which nursing task is (or will be) the easiest for you?

   _____

2. Which nursing task is (or will be) the most difficult for you?

   _____

3. What do you think is the most important duty you have?

   _____

4. What do you think is the least important duty you have?

_____

5. Who always lends you a hand?

_____

6. Who do you always lend a hand to?

_____

7. Who has gone to bat for you?

_____

8. Who have you gone to bat for?

_____

⇆ Communication Strategy

Referring to Others

Sometimes you want to help with a task, but you don't know how. It may be necessary to refer to others who have expertise or experience if you are not the appropriate person to ask. There are some specific phrases to use when doing this.

Phrases to refer to others

> I've never done that, but Nurse X has.
>
> I don't know how to do that, but Nurse X does.
>
> I'm not an expert in that. Maybe you should ask X.
>
> I've never heard of/seen that. Let's ask X.
>
> I know someone who can answer your question/who can help.
>
> This calls for someone with more experience than I have.
>
> The person who can help you is Nurse X.

Idioms to refer to others

> Nurse X is my point person.
>
> Nurse X is my go-to person.

⇆ Communication Strategy

Requesting and Giving Help

When health care workers ask someone to do something, they are making a request. Workers may ask supervisors, colleagues, or those they supervise for help. They must be sure to use the proper form before the verb when making a request. Most requests begin with a greeting, such as to say *hi* or *hello*. You can also **clear** your throat or give a non-verbal cue that you will be making a request.

Formal

Could/Can you please
Excuse me. Do you think that you could/can
I'm sorry to bother you. I wonder if you could/can
I wonder if you could/can
Pardon me. Could/Can you
Hi, Would you mind [help]ing

Informal

Help/Teach me
How about helping
I need you to
Tell me how to

When someone asks you to do something, you can respond positively or negatively. If you cannot help the person, you should give the reason why.

Positive responses

All right.	No problem.
Certainly.	Of course.
I'd be glad to.	O.K.
My pleasure.	Sure.

Negative responses

I'm afraid I can't.
I'd like to, but I can't.
I'm sorry. I can't.

Worker: Can you please teach me how to sterilize the door knobs?

Supervisor: I'm sorry. I can't. I need to go to the intensive care unit. Please ask Kristina to help you.

Dialogue Completion

Complete the dialogues using an appropriate response.

1. *Head Nurse:*   Would you mind clearing the halls? We need to remove the deceased from Room 211.

   Nurse: _____. (positive response)

2. *Doctor:*   Can you please take Mr. Natdar's vital signs?

   Nurse: _____. (positive response)

3. *Nurse:*   I need you to get some portable O_2 in here.

   Hospital Worker: _____. (positive response)

4. *New Nurse:*   Excuse me. Can you show me how to fill out this form?

   Registered Nurse: _____. (negative response)

5. *Family Member:*   I wonder if you could tell me how to get to the cafeteria?

   Nursing Assistant: _____. (positive response) Take the elevator to the ground floor, and then go left.

6. *New nurse:*   Sir, could you possibly recommend me for a promotion?

   Supervisor: _____. (negative response)

Dialogue Practice

Read and practice the dialogues with a partner.

1. *Doctor:*   Can you assist during the tracheotomy?

   New Nurse: I've never done one of those, but Nurse Richey has.

2. *Client:*   I'd like to know how to get information about nursing homes for my grandmother.

   Nurse: I'm new here, but I know someone who can tell you. I'll find her.

3. *Relative:*   My mother's wound actually seems worse today. What does that mean?

   Nursing Assistant: The person who can help you is Nurse Ying.

Referring

Write an appropriate answer to the questions, referring to nurses or people you know.

1. What do you know about triple bypass surgery?

    _____ .

2. This client only speaks Vietnamese. Is there a nurse here who can help?

    _____ .

3. Can you help me with my anxiety attacks here in the hospital?

    _____ .

⇆ Communication Strategy

Expressing *Thank You* and *You're Welcome*

After a health care worker helps someone, the person who made the request often expresses gratitude. There are many ways to say thanks, both formally or informally, depending on the situation. It is important to choose an appropriate term.

Formal
> I'm (very/so) grateful for your help.
> Thank you (so much) for your help.
> Thank you very much. I really appreciate it.

Less Formal
> That was nice of you. Thank you.
> Thank you. You really shouldn't have.

Informal
> Thanks.
> Thanks a lot.
> Thanks a million.

Respond to someone's gratitude with an appropriate phrase that means "you're welcome."

Formal
> You're (very/quite/more than) welcome.
> (It was) my pleasure.
> Don't mention it.
> Not at all.

Informal
> Anytime.
> Don't worry about it.
> Forget it.
> (It's) no big deal.
> (It's) no problem.
> Mm-hmm.
> Sure.

Dialogue Completion

Complete the dialogues using an appropriate response.

1. *New Nurse:*   Thank you. That was nice of you.

   Head Nurse: _____

2. *Nurse's Aide.*   Thanks a lot!

   Nurse.   _____

3. *Client's Husband:*   I'm so grateful for your help.

   Doctor: _____

4. *Nursing Assistant:*   Thanks! That was great advice.

   Nurse: _____

Situation Analysis

For each situation, discuss whether or not the person should say thanks. Discuss your reasons.

1. A nurse asks the client for his birth date to put on a form. The client gives the information.

   _____

2. A nurse takes a client's glasses from on top of a tray and puts them on the bedside table.

   _____

3. A nurse says to a client, "I'll be back in about 15 minutes."

   _____

Pronunciation: /sh/ and /ch/ Sounds

Each letter in the English alphabet has at least one individual sound, but sometimes two letters together make a new sound. The letters *s* and *c* are combined with the letter *h* to make new sounds.

Rule: The letters *s* and *h* combine to make the /sh/ sound and *c* and *h* make the /ch/ sound.

The /sh/ Sound

Read the words with the /sh/ sound with a partner.

1. shift	4. show	7. wash
2. shot	5. shoes	8. finish
3. shut	6. shower	9. gash

Sentences with the /sh/ Sound

Say *Show me how to* before each phrase.

1. . . . wash the wound.

2. . . . give a shot.

3. . . . shut this window.

4. . . . finish it.

5. . . . give the client a shower.

6. . . . shine my shoes.

The /ch/ Sound

Read the words with the /ch/ sound with a partner.

1. check	5. chart	9. teach
2. choose	6. discharge	10. lunch
3. child	7. kitchen	11. touch
4. chin	8. Achoo!	12. church

Sentences with the /ch/ Sound

Say *Nurse **Ch**en wants* . . . before each phrase.

1. . . . to **ch**eck her **ch**art.

2. . . . some **ch**ocolate.

3. . . . a new wat**ch**.

4. . . . to visit the kit**ch**en.

5. . . . to dis**ch**arge the client.

6. . . . to eat **ch**icken with **ch**eese for lun**ch**.

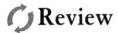 # Review

Dialogue Review

Review the dialogue on page 61. As you read, follow the directions. Then compare your answers with a partner.

- Underline the **Work** terms.
- Circle the **Requesting Help/Giving Help** phrases.
- Box the **Express Gratitude** phrases.

Role Plays: Helping with Tasks

Work with a partner. Read each situation, and develop a dialogue to perform for the class.

1. A first year nurse asks a supervisor to help her use a new kind of blood pressure cuff.

2. A nurse offers to lend a hand to another nurse who looks too busy. The second nurse accepts the help.

3. A supervisor shows a nurse's aide where to find clean towels.

4. A client thanks a doctor for saving his life.

5. A nurse asks another nurse to teach her how to say *Good morning* in a client's language. The second nurse refers her to someone who knows that language.

6. A nursing student wants to learn how to take a client's temperature. His professor shows him.

7. A busy nurse asks a colleague for help with some routine tasks.

Interacting in General

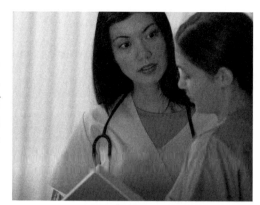

Health care workers communicate with each other throughout their shifts. The interaction is mostly face-to-face, but it may also happen on the telephone. If something is not clear, it is important to clarify the information. Health care workers also need to clarify information for clients.

Listening to the Action

Listening for Language

Listen to the conversations between health care workers and clients. What phrases do the clients use when they want to clarify something the health care workers say?

1. _____

2. _____

3. _____

⇅ Dialogue

Practicing the Language

The Maternity Ward nurses station is very busy with phone calls. Practice the dialogue in groups of three.

Nurse: Good evening. Dallas General Hospital Maternity Ward. This is Lu. How may I help you?

Caller 1: Yes, this is Dr. Sutton. I'd like to speak to Dr. Shank about a SIDS research study I'm doing.

Nurse: Dr. Shank is in the N.I.C.U. right now. I'll transfer you to that floor.

Caller 1: O.K. Thanks.

Nurse: Good evening. Dallas General Hospital Maternity Ward. This is Lu. May I help you?

Caller 2: Yes, I'm calling to find out if Zoe Cavanaugh has had her baby.

Nurse: Cava . . . ? How do you spell that, please?

Caller 2: C-a-v-a-n-a-u-g-h.

Nurse: I need to check and see. Hold on, please. [pause] Hello? Yes, she's had the babies and has already been discharged.

Caller 2: I'm sorry. Babies?

Nurse: Yes, she had twins.

$\overset{A\,B}{C}$ Vocabulary

Acronyms

An acronym is an abbreviation that is often pronounced as one word. *Scuba,* for example, is an acronym. *Scuba* stands for "**S**elf-**C**ontained **U**nderwater **B**reathing **A**pparatus," but we use it as a word. In English, you would see, "I will go scuba diving." You will not see, "I will go S.C.U.B.A. Diving." It is important to know which abbreviations are really acronyms so that you can pronounce them correctly.

There are acronyms for locations, illnesses, and procedures (or words associated with procedures). Most acronyms are created from the first letter of each word, but some are formed from more than one letter or from parts of each word. Some common acronyms are listed.

- **illnesses and conditions:** REM, AIDS, SARS, SAD, SIDS
- **procedure or procedure words:** LASIK, PIXELS, LASER, CAT

Learning Common Acronyms

Write the long version of each acronym.

1. AIDS _____

2. CAT _____

3. LASER _____

4. LASIK _____

5. PIXELS _____

6. REM _____

7. SAD _____

8. SARS _____

9. SIDS _____

10. ROM _____

Using Acronyms

Choose an acronym from the list on page 71, and then use it in an original sentence. The first one has been done for you as an example.

1. *LASIK surgery is now more common than in the past.*

2. _____ .

3. _____ .

4. _____ .

5. _____ .

⇆ Communication Strategy

Clarification Requests for Meaning

When you do not understand the meaning of a word that a person says, you can ask the person to explain or repeat it. There are three ways to do this.

Interrupt Politely and Repeat

I am sorry. SARS?

Pardon me. SARS?

Excuse me. SARS?

Ask for Spelling

SARS? How do you spell that?

Ask Directly

SARS? What does that mean?

Uh . . . I don't understand. Can you explain SARS?

Excuse me, what does SARS mean?

Dialogue Practice

Read and practice these dialogues with a partner.

1. *Supervising Nurse:* How is the client's SARS?

   Nursing Student: I am sorry. What does SARS mean?

   Supervising Nurse: Oh, it means Severe Acute Respiratory Syndrome.

   Nursing Student: I understand now, thank you. His SARS is responding to antibiotics.

2. *Nurse 1:* Are you going to have LASIK?

   Nurse 2: Uh. I don't understand. LASIK?

   Nurse 1: Yeah, the eye surgery.

   Nurse 2: Oh, thanks for explaining.

Practicing Clarification

Ask or tell your partner about the job you want to have. Your partner will use clarification requests. Then reverse roles.

⇄ Communication Strategy

Using the Telephone

Some health care workers need to answer the phone every day. Others only need to answer the phone once in a while. Either way, clear communication on the phone is important when a health care worker is talking to co-workers, supervisors, or the public while on the job. Answering the telephone requires four steps.

Step 1—Greetings
Good morning / Good afternoon / Good evening.

Step 2—Name of medical center and department
University Hospital—Pathology
University Hospital—I.C.U. Nursing Station
University Hospital—Cardiac Recovery

Step 3—Self-Identification
[Patty] speaking.
This is [Patty].

Step 4—Offer of Help
How may I direct your call?
How may I help you?
May I help you?

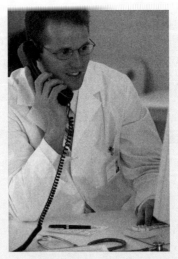

If a health care worker is unable to help the person on the phone, instead of taking a message, he or she will most likely try to find someone to help. In this case, the staff member needs to put the caller on hold. There are several ways to do this.

Formal
Do you mind if I put you on hold?
I need to ask about that.
May I put you on hold?
Would you mind holding?

Less Formal
Could/Can you hold, please?
Will you hold, please?
I need to check and see.

Informal
Hold on, please.
I'm going to put you on hold.

Sometimes you will have to transfer a call to someone else. You can do this formally or informally.

Formal
I'll transfer you to the Chief Nursing Officer, who will be able to help you.

Less Formal
I'll put you through to the Chief Nursing Officer, who will be able to help you.

Informal
I'll connect you with the Chief Nursing Officer. He'll help you.

Writing Dialogues

Write responses for answering the telephone from the areas of a medical center. Use different phrases from the list on page 74. Then read your responses to a partner. The first one has been done for you as an example.

1. Maternity Check-In

   "Good morning. University Hospital—Maternity Check-In. This is Anton. How may I help you?"

2. Pediatrics

   _____

3. 5th floor Nursing Station

   _____

4. Med-Psych Unit

   _____

5. Radiology

   _____

6. Center for Pain Management

   _____

7. Physical Therapy

   _____

8. Breast Cancer Clinic

   _____

9. Oncology Nursing Station

   _____

10. Emergency Department

    _____

Dialogue Completion

Complete the dialogues with an appropriate phrase from the box on page 74. Then read and practice them with a partner.

1. *Nurse:* Good afternoon. University Hospital—Outpatient Surgery.

   _____. _____.

   Caller: Yes, I'm scheduled for a procedure tomorrow, but I won't be able to make it. There's been a death in the family.

   Nurse: Oh, I'm sorry to hear that. _____.
   They will be able to re-schedule you.

2. *Nurse:* _____. University Hospital—Maternity.

   _____. _____?

   Caller: Hi. I'm trying to locate my sister. I think that she may have been taken to this hospital. Her baby's not due until next month, but I got a message that an ambulance came to pick her up.

   Nurse: What's your sister's name?

   Caller: Kelly Saluski.

   Nurse: O.K. _____.

   Caller: Yes.

   (caller holds)

   Nurse: Miss? Yes, she's here and the baby is, too! She's in the I.C.U. _____.
   They'll be able to give you more information.

Pronunciation: /th/, /ph/, and /gh/ Sounds

In English, there are many combined sounds. The letters *t, p,* and *g* can be combined with *h*.

   Rule: The letters *t* and *h* combine to make the /th/ sound. The letters *p* and *g* combine with *h* to make the /f/ sound.

The /th/ Sound

Read the words with the /th/ sound with a partner.

1. think	5. nothing	9. teeth
2. thank	6. something	10. month
3. thirsty	7. anesthetic	11. mouth
4. thin	8. catheter	12. bath

Sentences with the /th/ Sound

Say I **th**ink before each phrase.

    1. . . . it's **Th**ursday.

    2. . . . he needs his ba**th**.

    3. . . . she's **th**irsty.

    4. . . . some**th**ing is wrong with the ca**th**.

    5. . . . it's next mon**th**.

    6. . . . he's very **th**in.

The /f/ Sound

Read the words with the /f/ sound with a partner.

    1. **ph**otogra**ph**   5. lau**gh**

    2. tele**ph**one   6. enou**gh**

    3. **ph**armacy   7. cou**gh**

    4. ne**ph**ew   8. rou**gh**

Sentences with the /f/ Sound

Say Dr. **Ph**ilippe . . . before each phrase.

    1. . . . lau**gh**s a lot.

    2. . . . has a cou**gh**.

    3. . . . called the **ph**armacy.

    4. . . . talks on the **ph**one.

    5. . . . can be tou**gh**.

    6. . . . likes to take **ph**otos.

Spelling

Fill in the blanks with the letters *th, sh, ch, ph,* or *gh.* Then check your answers with a partner.

1. mou __ __ wa __ __

2. __ __ eck his __ __ art

3. tou __ __ job

4. painful to tou __ __

5. __ __ one call

6. __ __ arp knife

7. bad cou __ __

8. __ __ ank you

9. family __ __ oto

10. __ __ ower and __ __ ampoo

11. tee __ __ in a mou __ __

12. dis __ __ arge the __ __ ild

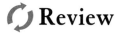 Review

Dialogue Review

Review the dialogue on page 75. As you read, follow the directions. Then compare your answers with a partner.

- Underline the **Acronyms.**
- Circle the **Clarification Request for Meaning.**
- Box the **Using the Telephone** phrases.

Role Plays: General Interaction between Colleagues

Work with a partner. Read each situation, and develop a dialogue to perform for the class.

1. One nurse's aide doesn't know what MODS (multi-organ dysfunction syndrome) means. A colleague explains.

2. A person calls the hospital pharmacy and asks if she can buy medical marijuana.

3. A client is confused by CAT and C.T. and asks a nurse to clarify.

4. A nurse in the emergency department receives a call, puts the caller on hold, and then transfers the call to the chaplain's office.

5. A client speaks to a doctor about his SARS and asks the doctor to clarify the meaning of SARS.

6. A nurse answers the phone and deals with a panicked relative.

7. A client overhears the word LASER and asks a nursing assistant how to spell it.

End-of-Unit Discussion

Sharing

Discuss the questions with a small group.

1. Is it better to try to help, even if you don't exactly know how, or to refer someone to another person?

2. Why is it necessary for a health care workers to be assertive?

3. What are some techniques to memorize acronyms?

4. Why is it important to get to know your co-workers well? How can that help during your day-to-day work?

Culture Point: Saying No

Read this story. Discuss in small groups and as a class.

————

Amber was unhappy that the parking garage that hospital employees use was raising their daily rate. She was planning to ask the CEO of the hospital to go to bat for the employees and bargain for a lower fee. She has prepared a petition and asked for other workers to sign.

Amber:	Hi, Satoko, can you sign my petition for reduced parking rates?
Satoko:	Maybe.
Amber:	Oh, please? I need everyone to sign it!
Satoko:	O.K.

Amber left the petition with Satoko, but was surprised to see it back in her mailbox unsigned.

————

Why did Satoko say "O.K." to Amber?

UNIT 5: Working with Doctors and Supervisors

All health care workers have a supervisor. Each day workers interact with their doctors and supervisors. They solve problems together. The language health care workers use with supervisors is more formal than the language they use with colleagues. It is important to use the appropriate phrases when talking to a supervisor.

Understanding Others on the Job

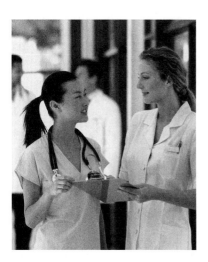

On the job, communication between health care workers and their supervisors is usually very focused (specific). There is not a lot of time for other conversation. Also, the rate of speech may be very quick. Communication must be clear. The health care worker must not hesitate to ask for clarification or confirmation of important orders or information.

Listening to the Action

 Listening for Language

Listen to the conversations between health care workers and supervisors. What phrases do the health care workers use to confirm information?

1. _____

2. _____

3. _____

⇅ Dialogue

Practicing the Language

It's a busy day. Doctors and nurses at Mercy Hospital are dealing with clients being transferred from the site of a train crash. They set up a triage area in the hallway near the emergency entrance. The Chief Nursing Officer (CNO) is deciding which clients have the most serious injuries. Practice the dialogue in groups of seven.

Chief Nursing Officer:	How much room do they have in the ED?
Nurse 1:	Not much. Only for those worst off.
Chief Nursing Officer:	[examining a client] Pupils are constricted. Heart rate is 120 . . . 110. . . . Get the defibrillator. Clear! [uses the defibrillator] Get this one into a trauma bay now!
Nurse 1:	Yes, right away.
Chief Nursing Officer:	[talking to a client] Hey, buddy. Can you hear me? [client blacks out] Nurse! Nurse! Get this one into the ED, STAT!
Nurse 2:	I'm on it.
Client:	Help me!
Chief Nursing Officer:	Tell me where it hurts.
Client:	My [inaudible]'s broken.
Chief Nursing Officer:	Can you repeat? What's broken?
Client:	My arm. My arm's broken.
Chief Nursing Officer:	Hang on. We'll get a nurse here to help you as soon as we can. [goes to help another client] This one's got head trauma. Line him up for the ED. Nurse; we're going to need about 50 units of blood. Call the lab.
Nurse 3:	Please clarify the number—15 or 50?
Chief Nursing Officer:	50!
Nurse 3:	Got it.
Emergency Medical Technician:	[wheeling in another client] This one's beyond help.
Chief Nursing Officer:	[examines client] You're right. We need someone to call it.
Nurse 4:	[looks at clock] The time of death is 4:04 PM.

Vocabulary

Words about a Serious Illness or Injury

There are specific phrases to use when a person has a serious illness or has been badly injured. These phrases are used in the ED and in other areas of a hospital.

- **Phrases to Describe Serious Illness or Injury:** a degenerative disease, in cardiac arrest, in declining health, in trauma, on life support
- **Idioms:** to black out, to call it (the time of death), worse off, the worst off

---

Matching

Match the phrases in the left column with the best description in the right column.

1. in declining health _____   a. losing consciousness

2. a degenerative disease _____   b. having a heart attack

3. in trauma _____   c. the person's health is getting worse and worse

4. in cardiac arrest _____   d. condition is bad compared to others

5. to black out _____   e. having a serious physical injury or is in shock

6. worse off _____   f. living because a machine is helping someone breathe

7. on life support _____   g. stating the time of death

8. to call it _____   h. an illness that makes a person sicker and sicker

---

Dialogue Completion

Complete these dialogues using the phrases given. Then practice with a partner.

1. *Nursing Professor:* Clients coming to the ED _____ get immediate medical attention.

   Nursing Student: That means they've had a severe accident or were victims of violence, right?

2. *Surgeon 1:* We lost him. I need you _____.

   Surgeon 2: The time of death is 10:30 AM.

3. *Nursing Aide:* The client in 401-B appears to be a lot sicker this week than last week.

   Nursing Supervisor: Yes, she is _____.

4. *Doctor:* Please call Mrs. Devine's family to the hospital since we may have to put her _____ tonight.

   Nurse: Right away.

Sentence Completion

Complete the sentences to show that you understand the meaning of the phrases being used. The first one has been done for you as an example.

1. The teenager blacked out _____*after being in the sun too long*_____.

2. Clients must be put on life support _____.

3. The business executive was in cardiac arrest _____ _____.

4. A client who has _____ is worse off than a client who has _____.

5. _____ is a degenerative disease.

⇄ Communication Strategy

Repetition Requests

When you do not hear or understand what a person says, you can ask them to say it again. There are formal and informal ways to do this. You must be careful to use the appropriate form when making a request.

Formal

I am sorry. Would you mind saying that again, please?

Pardon me/Excuse me. Could/Can you repeat that, please?

<u>Note</u>: If there is an emergency, these forms can be shorter (e.g., "Repeat, please!")

Less Formal

Could you say that again?

I didn't get that. Can you say it again?

I didn't understand what you said.

Can you please clarify?

Informal

What was that?

Come again?

Say again?

I'm sorry?

Dialogue Practice

Read and practice the dialogues with a partner.

1. *Supervisor:* Can you check Storeroom 2 for the missing syringes?

   Nurse: Pardon me. Could you repeat that, please?

   Supervisor: Check Storeroom 2 to look for the missing syringes.

   Nurse: Yes, sir. Right away.

2. *Relative:* I think my brother's gonna croak!

   Nursing Assistant: I didn't understand what you said.

   Relative: My brother was shot. I think he's going to die!

3. *Nurse 1:* I am taking tomorrow off!

   Nurse 2: Did you get approval from the supervisor?

   Nurse 1: What was that?

   Nurse 2: Did you ask the supervisor?

   Nurse 1: Uh. Uhm. No, not yet.

Dialogue Completion

Complete the dialogues. Choose appropriate repetition requests from the box on page 83.

1. *Doctor:* Can you relay the results of his biopsy to Mr. Alwakeel's family members?

   You: _____

2. *One of your classmates:* Help me prep for the test?

   You: _____

3. *Hospital Administrator:* Make sure that this equipment is in tip-top shape before the inspection.

   You: _____

4. *Nurse:* The client in 208-A is complaining of back pain.

   You: _____

5. *Client:* Can you tell the kitchen that I don't want any more gelatin for dessert?

   You: _____

⇆ Communication Strategy

Agreeing

Sometimes you have the same opinion, idea, or emotion as another person. You can agree with what he or she says. There are many ways to agree with someone, and there are some common phrases that are used for agreeing.

Formal

> I agree.
> That's/You're right.
> You make a good point.

Informal

> I think so too.
> Absolutely.
> Definitely.
> For sure.
> How true.
> You can say that again!

Dialogue Completion

Complete the dialogues with an appropriate phrase from the box. Then read and practice the dialogues with a partner.

1. *Nurse:*   He appears to have severe allergies.

   Doctor: _____.

2. *Client:*   I think I'll be well enough to go home soon.

   Nurse: _____.

3. *Nurse 1:*   That was one of the busiest shifts I've had this year!

   Nurse 2:   _____.

4. *Nurse:*   Could you please repeat?

   Supervisor: We're going to need to contact the next of kin.

   Nurse: _____.

Writing Dialogues

Read the topics, and write dialogues in which one person gives an opinion and the other agrees with it. The first one has been done for you as an example.

1. Stress on the job

   A: I think _our jobs can be very stressful._

   B: How true.

2. Pediatric patients

   A: I think _____.

   B: _____.

3. Understanding doctor's orders

   A: I think _____.

   B: _____.

4. Asking for a promotion

   A: I think _____.

   B: _____.

5. The food in the cafeteria

   A: I think _____.

   B: _____.

Pronunciation: Stress in Numbers

Most confusion with numbers from 1 to 100 in English is due to the stress in pronunciation. You must carefully pronounce the teen and ten numbers.

Rule: The teen numbers have the stress on the syllable containing *teen,* and the *t* sound is very clear. The ten numbers that end in *–ty* have the stress on the first syllable, and the *t* in *–ty* sounds like a *d* (not a *t*).

Pronouncing Numbers

Read the numbers two times. First, read them vertically. Then read them horizontally. Make sure to stress the syllable with the stress.

13	thirteen	30	thirty
14	fourteen	40	forty
15	fifteen	50	fifty
16	sixteen	60	sixty
17	seventeen	70	seventy
18	eighteen	80	eighty
19	nineteen	90	ninety

Recognizing Numbers

Listen to your instructor read one sentence from each pair. Mark the sentence you hear. Then practice this exercise with a partner.

1. _____ Room 815 needs to be cleaned.

   _____ Room 850 needs to be cleaned.

2. _____ About 14 EMTs arrived at the site of the plane crash.

   _____ About 10 EMTs arrived at the site of the plane crash.

3. _____ There are 19 people in the waiting room.

   _____ There are 90 people in the waiting room.

4. _____ Respirator 13 is out of order.

   _____ Respirator 30 is out of order.

5. _____ Admitting requires 18 forms.

   _____ Admitting requires 80 forms.

6. _____ A 17-year-old will get a lung transplant later today.

   _____ A 70-year-old will get a lung transplant later today.

7. _____ Bus 16 goes directly to the hospital from here.

   _____ Bus 60 goes directly to the hospital from here.

8. _____ The most expensive gift in the gift shop costs $15 dollars.

   _____ The most expensive gift in the gift shop costs $50 dollars.

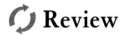 # Review

Dialogue Review

Review the dialogue on page 81. As you read, follow the directions. Then compare your answers with a partner.

- Underline the **Serious Illness or Injury** terms.
- Circle the **Repetition Requests**.
- Box the **Agreement** phrase.

Role Plays: Understanding Others on the Job

Work with a partner. Read each situation, and develop a dialogue to perform for the class.

1. The charge nurse is talking to a nurse at the beginning of a shift. The charge nurse is listing the room numbers of the most seriously ill clients on the fourth floor. The nurse needs to take notes.

2. A nursing student is assisting a doctor who is taking care of a broken arm. The student doesn't understand the word *pins* in this case.

3. A Human Resources staff member calls a new employee to say that his hospital badge number has been changed.

4. A nurse is telling a nurse's aide all the things that must be done on the shift.

5. The staff psychologist gives a phone number to a visitor. The visitor is elderly and can't hear well.

6. A staff nutritionist is explaining to a client what can and cannot be eaten after being discharged. The client is taking notes and asks a lot of questions.

7. A client who had severe head trauma dies. A doctor asks for someone to call the time of death.

Interacting with Supervisors

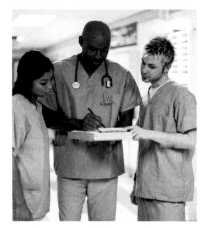

Health care workers spend a lot of time with their supervisors. In order to do a good job, communication must be clear. It is difficult to learn every new task or skill the first time it is introduced. It is necessary to ask questions to understand all the details. If the information is given over the phone, it is even more important to make sure everything is clear. If you make a mistake or do something incorrectly, you can apologize.

Listening to the Action

 Listening for Language

Listen to the conversations between health care workers and supervisors. What specific phrases do the health care workers use to apologize?

1. _____

2. _____

3. _____

⇕ Dialogue

Practicing the Language

It's a busy day for a nurse who has just graduated and started working at Good Samaritan Hospital. The nurse learns that it is not always easy to understand what a supervisor wants or needs. Practice the dialogue in pairs.

Supervisor: How's everything today?

Nurse: Fine. We're busy, but everything's fine.

Supervisor: Did you finish checking your meds?

Nurse: No, not yet. I haven't gotten around to it yet.

Supervisor: Have you taken vitals already this morning?

Nurse: I'll be done with that in a few minutes. Can I ask question about bed pans and bed baths? Can I always ask a CNA to do those?

Supervisor: Always? Hmmm. No, not always. Sometimes you need to do them yourself.

Nurse: Oh, my fault, then. I thought that there would be enough CNAs to help with that. That's what we learned at nursing school.

Supervisor: Well, every hospital is different.

Nurse: I find that I'm getting a handle on some things but missing the point on others.

Supervisor: I think that you are going to figure everything out soon.

Nurse: That's good to hear. I'm sorry to ask so many questions.

Supervisor: Sorry? No worries. Asking questions is a sign of a good nurse.

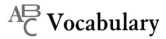 Vocabulary

Idioms Associated with Understanding and Not Understanding

While you are in training or on the job, you are learning new skills and procedures. Sometimes the instructions are very detailed and you may not understand right away. Your supervisor may use these phrases or idioms with you or you may use these phrases to describe if you understand or do not understand.

- **Understand:** to catch on, to figure (something) out, to get a handle on/to get the hang of, to get it, to have a knack for, to put two and two together

  <u>Note</u>: All the phrases in the list can also be negative.

  I don't get it.

- **Do not understand:** (something) goes in one ear and out the other, (something) goes over someone's head, is beyond + [object pronoun] (*That's beyond me!*), is Greek to + [object pronoun] (*That's Greek to me!*), to miss the point, to not make heads or tails (of something)

Using the Negative

Rewrite the sentences so they are negative.

1. They get a handle on things quickly. _____

2. She's gotten the hang of things. _____

3. I can catch on. _____

4. I can put two and two together. _____

5. He can figure it out. _____

6. You have a knack for that. _____

Sentence Completion

Complete the sentences to show that you understand the meaning of the idioms being used. The first one has been done for you as an example.

1. I can't make heads or tails of _*what that doctor says.*_____

2. I missed the point when the supervisor talked about _____.

3. _____ is beyond me.

4. For me, how to _____ goes in one ear and out the other.

5. _____ went over my head.

Choosing the Correct Preposition

Complete the sentences with appropriate prepositions.

1. I couldn't make heads _____ tails of that new ventilator.

2. Katia always catches _____ more quickly than others.

3. Can you figure _____ what the supervisor told us about the breathing equipment?

4. I'm tired today. Everything seems to go _____ one ear and _____ the other.

5. On his first day on the job, the doctor's orders went _____ his head. That's why the client got the wrong meal tray.

6. They tried to teach us how to fix a malfunctioning heart pump, but it was all Greek _____ me.

⇆ Communication Strategy

Responding

At times supervisors will ask you how you are doing. They usually want to know about the progress of your work. There are ways to make this clear. Sometimes you need to tell them that the work is not done yet. Other times you need to tell them when the work will be done.

Responding when work is not done yet
I'll be done in a minute.
I'm doing the best I can.
I'm working on it.
It may take a while.
It shouldn't be long.
It'll just be a second.
It'll only take another second.

Responding when work has not been started yet
I haven't gotten around to it yet.
I'll do it later.
I'll get to it soon / later / tomorrow.
I'll have it ready soon / later / tomorrow.
I'll see what I can do.
It should be no problem.

Dialogue Practice

Read and practice the dialogue with a partner.

Supervisor: How is it going? Have you finished your task yet?

Nurse: I'm working on it.

Supervisor: When will it be done?

Nurse: It shouldn't be long.

Supervisor: When!

Nurse: I'll have it ready by the end of the shift.

Supervisor: O.K. That's fine.

Dialogue Completion

Complete the dialogues with an appropriate response from the box on page 92.

1. *Supervisor:*   Did you dispose of the contaminated bandages yet?

   Nurse's Aide: _____.

2. *Administrator:*   Will you send out the memo soon?

   Nurse: _____.

3. *Nurse:*   Can we get a bigger supply of thermometers at the nurse's station?

   Staff Member: _____.

4. *Nurse 1:*   When can you have that chart updated?

   Nurse 2:   _____.

5. *Client:*   Are you getting my pills ready? I need my pills, you know.

   Nurse's Aide: _____.

Dialogue Analysis

Read and practice the dialogues with a partner. Then answer the questions.

1. *A:* Why haven't you checked on the new client yet?

   B: I'm doing the best I can!

2. *A:* Are you going to be able to get a birthday cake for me tomorrow?

   B: I'll see what I can do.

3. *A:* How long are you going to keep that needle in me?

   B: It'll just take a second.

- Who is A? Who is B?
- Where are they?
- Can you expand the dialogue and use another responding strategy?

⇆ Communication Strategy

Apologizing

If you make a mistake on the job, you need to take responsibility and apologize. You should also apologize if you hurt or bother someone. There are various phrases you can say to show that you feel bad about your actions. Apologizing can be formal or informal, depending on the situation. Use the appropriate form, and explain your actions when possible.

Formal

> My apologies.
> Please accept my apologies.
> Please excuse/forgive me.

Less Formal

> I apologize.
> I'm really/so/very sorry.

Informal

> Oops!
> Sorry.
> Sorry about that.

The supervisor who receives a formal apology may formally accept it. In informal situations, some people and some cultures sometimes do not accept apologies simply because they do not want to feel superior or to make the other person feel badly. If they do not directly accept the apology, they usually try to respond somehow.

Responses

> Don't worry about it.
> No problem.
> No worries.
> That's all right.
> That's O.K.

Dialogue Practice

Read and practice the dialogues with a partner.

1. *Nurse:*   I'm sorry to keep you waiting.

   Elderly Client: Yeah. I have been waiting for more than 30 minutes.

   Nurse: I apologize. I was helping someone else.

   Elderly Client: O.K. Well, I would like to have my bath now.

   Nurse: No problem.

2. *Nurse 1:*   Hey, you forgot to bring me those supplies.

   Nurse 2:   Oops!

   Nurse 1:   I really need them.

   Nurse 2:   Sorry. I'll go get them right now.

Writing Apologies

Write an appropriate apology. Then read them with a partner.

1. You spilled water on a client.

   _____

2. You gave a co-worker the wrong towels to use.

   _____

3. You forgot it was your co-worker's birthday.

   _____

4. You have been late to work every day for two weeks.

   _____

5. You didn't understand what a teenage client is saying.

   _____

Pronunciation: Intonation to Show Surprise

When we are surprised at something we hear, our voice changes. Listen to your instructor read the sentence. Does the statement of surprise have rising (↗) or falling (↘) intonation?

You ate five bananas!?

Rule: When expressing surprise, use rising intonation (↗).

Expressing Surprise

Listen and repeat the sentences using rising intonation with a partner. Then read the statements again, and change the underlined word to a new word.

1. She has 18 children!?

2. You saw the President of the United States in the lobby!?

3. The client swallowed a pearl necklace!?

4. A chicken ran into the ED!?

5. You only sleep for five hours!?

6. What!?

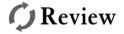# Review

Dialogue Review

Review the dialogue on page 90. As you read, follow the directions. Then compare your answers with a partner.

- Underline the **Idioms for Understanding or Not Understanding**.
- Circle the **Responding Strategies**.
- Box the **Ways to Apologize**.

Role Plays: Interacting with Supervisors

Work with a partner. Read each situation, and develop a dialogue to perform for the class.

1. A supervisor praises a new nurse about how well he has learned all of the policies and procedures of the job.

2. A nursing student is rushing through a hallway and bumps into one of the medical directors and formally apologizes.

3. A supervisor asks a nursing assistant if she has transferred the clients to the new rooms. The assistant uses a responding strategy.

4. A nurse apologizes to a client after spilling some water when putting the cup on the bed tray.

5. A nurse is surprised to hear that some members of a wedding party have just been admitted with food poisoning. When she asks how many, the answer is seven.

6. A nursing student is worried that she's not getting the hang of things as quickly as her classmates. She talks to her professor about this.

7. A nurse practitioner asks at the nursing station if they have called the pharmacy for missing medications. The nurse there uses a responding strategy.

End-of-Unit Discussion

Sharing

Discuss the questions with a small group.

1. Do you feel nervous when you ask others to repeat information? How can you gain more confidence as you are learning to be a health care worker and improving your English at the same time?

2. Which do you think are the worst diseases? Tell your classmates about them.

3. Some things are easy to learn and other things are harder to learn. Name one thing that you have caught onto quickly and one thing that keeps going over your head.

4. Which phrase do you prefer to use when you apologize? Which phrase do you prefer to use when you respond to an apology?

Culture Point: Working under Supervision

Read this story. Discuss in small groups and as a class.

Jeanne worked as a nursing assistant at Rose Medical Center. A new nursing assistant, Priva, just started. Priva's supervisor told her what to do and mentioned that Jeanne would be a good person to ask if she had any questions. On the second day of work, Priva talked to Jeanne . . .

Priva: How do you think I'm doing?

Jeanne: You're doing fine. You are catching on very quickly.

Priva: Where is our supervisor?

Jeanne: Well, she's usually busy, but she may check on us later in the day.

Priva: Oh??

Why was Priva surprised?

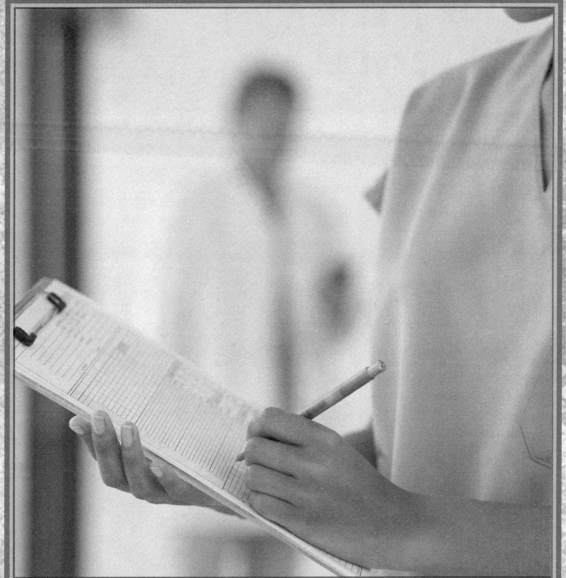

PART 3

Client Information

UNIT 6: Maintaining Client Records

In addition to physically caring for clients, health care workers must precisely document everything that is done. From the time the client is admitted to the facility to the time the client is discharged (and even after that), all assessments, interventions, consulting, or any other actions must be documented in writing. In addition to maintaining a client's chart, other forms such as Activities of Daily Living checklists or discharge forms must be completed and maintained.

Charting

Charting requires a large portion of time during a health care worker's shift. Charting is the act of documenting (electronically or by hand) a client's condition in the client's record (official document). The correct charting procedure in one medical facility may be incorrect in another. Therefore, it is important to ask enough questions to make sure that the charting information is clear and understood.

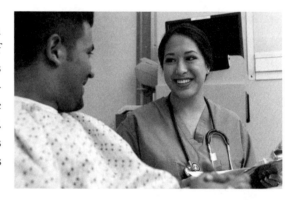

Listening to the Action

 Listening for Language

Listen to the conversations between an instructor and a nursing student. What does the student say to show that she understands?

1. _____

2. _____

3. _____

⇅ Dialogue

Practicing the Language

Some nursing students are reviewing some abbreviations with one of their instructors. Practice the dialogue in groups of four.

Student 1: So, we'll have a quiz on 15 abbreviations each week, is that correct?

Professor: Yes, on your handout the abbreviations are in alphabetical order, but you should study them in different ways, too.

Student 2: The most difficult ones are the ones that come from Latin. For example, P.O. means "by mouth" but comes from *per os,* right?

Professor: Yes, and N.P.O. means . . . ?

Student 2: Nothing by mouth.

Professor: Correct. Learn all of the abbreviations related to "manner" in a group. You know, P.O., N.P.O., P.R., I.V., I.M., or S.L.

Student 1: Can you explain why some abbreviations are pronounced like words, like STAT?

Professor: That kind of abbreviation is just a short form of a word, just like Kat can be a short form of Katherine.

Student 3: Can you tell us why some abbreviations have a slash? Like R/O?

Professor: No, I can't. That's just random.

ABC Vocabulary

Abbreviations

Abbreviations are standard in charting. When charting, abbreviations make the work go faster. Some abbreviations are universal, some are specific to the health care professions, and others may be approved, unique abbreviations for your workplace. When you write anything by hand, your handwriting must be very clear so that no mistakes are made. For example, 10 mgs must not look like 70 mgs.

Remember that the difference between an abbreviation and an acronym is that acronyms are pronounced as one word, but abbreviations are pronounced letter by letter. We have added periods between the letters to help you understand the difference.

There are common medical abbreviations related to time, manner, and place as well as some other general uses.

- **Time:** a.c., A.S.A.P., B.I.D., T.A., p.c., P.R.N., Q.I.D., T.I.D.

- **Manner:** I.M., I.V., N.P.O., P.O., P.R., S.L.

- **Place:** C.C.U., E.D./E.R., I.C.U., O.R., R.R.

- **Miscellaneous:** A.D.L., B.M., B.P., D.N.R., E.K.G., H.R., P.T., R/O

- **Locations:** P.I.C.U., M.I.C.U., N.I.C.U., I.C.U.

Defining Abbreviations

Write what each of the abbreviations represents. Then work with a group to explain the abbreviations to someone who is not a health care worker. The first one has been done for you as an example.

1. B.M. _bowel movement, A bowel movement is when excrement (or feces) passes through_ _the intestines and comes out of the body._

2. a.c. _____

3. A.D.L. _____

4. B.P. _____

5. C.C.U. _____

6. D.N.R. _____

7. E.D./E.R. _____

8. E.K.G. _____

9. E.T.A. _____

10. g.t.t.s. _____

11. I.C.U. _____

12. I.M. _____

13. I.V. _____

14. N.P.O. _____

15. O.R. _____

16. p.c. _____

17. P.O. _____

18. P.R. _____

19. P.T. _____

20. R/O _____

21. R.R. _____

22. S.L. _____

23. T.I.D. _____

Dialogue Practice

Read and practice the dialogues with a partner.

1. *Client:*   Is it possible to see my doctor soon?

    Nurse: He's in the ED. Maybe later.

    Client: Eating Disorder?!

    Nurse: No, the Emergency Department. ED is used for both of those things.

2. *Student Nurse 1:* Why are abbreviations so complicated! Why are a.c. and p.c. "before meals" and "after meals"? Why isn't it b.m. and a.m.?

    Student Nurse 2: Because B.M. is "bowel movement" and a.m. is "morning"! No, seriously . . . so many of the abbreviations come from Latin words. We just have to memorize them.

3. *Nurse's Aide 1:* How in the world is g.t.t.s. the abbreviation for "drops"?

    Nurse's Aide 2: I have no idea.

Adding More Abbreviations

Think of other common abbreviations that you are familiar with. List them, and write their meanings. Then share them with the class.

Abbreviation   Meaning

_____ _____

_____ _____

_____ _____

_____ _____

_____ _____

⇆ Communication Strategy

Confirmation Checks

When you need to make it clear (confirm) that you understand what someone says, you can repeat the main subject then add a phrase. There are various phrases to use. Add a question after the confirmation when someone is telling you very important information such as times or amounts. Use the other checks for less important information.

Confirming important information

_____, (is that) right?

_____, (am I) correct?

Confirming other information

_____, I understand.

_____, I got it.

_____, O.K.

Dialogue Practice

Read and practice the dialogues with a partner.

1. *Supervisor:* Mr. Lindley must not have any liquids after midnight.

   New Nurse: No liquids after midnight, I understand.

   Supervisor: And he must be ready for surgery at 8:00 AM.

   New Nurse: 8:00 AM, is that correct?

   Supervisor: Yes.

2. *Doctor:* Give him 500 mg of his medication every six hours.

   Nurse: Every six hours, right?

   Doctor: Yes, and make sure that the kitchen switches his meals to no salt.

   Nurse: No salt meals. I got it.

3. *Nurse 1:* Note that Mr. Trivoli has had an allergic reaction to eggs.

   Nurse 2: Allergic to eggs, O.K. Anything else?

   Nurse 1: Yes, the doctor wants him to be tested for diabetes.

   Nurse 2: Diabetes test, O.K.

Practicing Confirmations

Read the sentences. Then write the most important information on the line, and add a confirmation check. The first one has been done for you as an example.

1. The dosage needs to be increased to 1,000 mgs.

   <u>1,000 mgs.</u> _____, <u>is that right?</u> _____

2. She has been admitted complaining of chest pains and dizziness.

   _____, _____

3. This client has requested to sign a Do Not Resuscitate form.

   _____, _____

4. Her breathing has become more labored over the last few hours.

   _____, _____

5. He responds better to the treatment if his wife is in the room with him.

   _____, _____

6. A Code Blue was called on Mr. Shephard at about 4:30 P.M.

   _____, _____

Charting Comprehension Checks

Give some important information that needs to be charted to your partner. Your partner will repeat the main part and add a comprehension check. If your partner answers correctly, say, *Yes, that's right* or *O.K.*

Partner A's statements:

1. Increase the frequency to once every two hours.

2. His vitals have been stable over this shift.

3. Mrs. Hopkins ate three-fourths of her dinner.

4. The doctor has said that the cause of death was a massive heart attack.

Partner B's statements:

1. He is reporting an increase in pain in his upper back.

2. Johnny will be discharged tomorrow at 2:00 PM. if all goes well tonight.

3. Give him one aspirin along with his other medications.

4. The respiratory therapist needs to be scheduled for Shawn Kennedy tomorrow.

⇆ Communication Strategy

Soliciting Information

If something in a client's chart or on a form is not clear or does not seem complete, it is important for you to solicit or ask for more information. There are certain phrases you can use to do this.

This says ___ _____. What does that mean?

I'd like to know what this means.

Could / Can you explain _____?

Could / Can you explain how to _____?

This says _____. Could / Can you give an example of that?

Could / Can you tell me why it says to do this?

What kind of _____?

Dialogue Practice

Read and practice the dialogues with a partner.

1. *Nurse 1:*   I read that Mr. Kato needs help when ambulating. Can you explain how to do that?

   Nurse 2:   Yes, give him a walker, but stay by his side to make sure he doesn't let go of it. Go slow. Start with two walks to the end of the hall today.

2. *Nursing Student:*   This says, "1 tablet Q.I.D.? What does Q.I.D. mean?

   Professor: Q.I.D. means four times a day.

3. *Nurse's Aide:*   The client orders say to change the dressing. What kind of dressing pads does this wound need?

   Supervisor: Use the largest ones we have.

Solicitating Information

Write two ways to solicit information for the notes in a client's chart.

1. Her main problem is activity intolerance.

   a. _____.

   b. _____.

2. Reinforce the need for him to increase his fluid intake.

   a. _____.

   b. _____.

3. His initial diagnosis is R/O TB.

   a. _____.

   b. _____.

4. Notify doctor if temperature is elevated.

   a. _____.

   b. _____.

Pronunciation: Stress in Abbreviations and Numbers

Abbreviations with three or more letters and numbers with three or four digits need to be carefully pronounced. Listen to your instructor read the examples. What letters or numbers are stressed?

He needs an E.K.G.

626-577-1224 (six two six, five seven seven, one two two four)

Rule: Most of the time, the first and last letters in an abbreviation are stressed. The first and last numbers in a small group of numbers are stressed.

Stress in Abbreviations and Numbers

Read the sentences, mark the appropriate stress, and then practice with a partner.

1. The phone number is 212-555-4624.

2. The client is in Room 1404, not Room 1440.

3. Tonight the I.C.U. is busier than the C.C.U.

4. His hospital employee number is 438-D117.

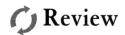 # Review

Dialogue Review

Review the dialogue on page 101. As you read, follow the directions. Then compare your answers with a partner.

- Underline the **Common Medical Abbreviations**.
- Circle the **Confirmation Checks**.
- Box the **Solicit Information** phrases.

Role Plays: Charting

Work with a partner. Read each situation, and develop a dialogue to perform for the class.

1. A nurse coming on shift doesn't understand an abbreviation on a chart and asks a supervisor about it.

2. A staff member in Admitting marks a new client as M (male) instead of F (female). The first nurse to interact with the client talks to the staff member.

3. A student nurse tells a supervisor that a client's "bag thingie" seems to be broken. The supervisor teaches the nurse about I.V.s.

4. A surgeon asks an anesthesiologist to explain something handwritten in a client's chart that was not clear.

5. A client tells a nurse about her special needs at dinnertime and the nurse responds with a confirmation check (so that it can be charted correctly).

6. A new nurse's aide doesn't clearly distinguish between the pronunciation of E.R., O.R., and R.R. The nurse charting the information writes the wrong room.

7. A client seems to have trouble seeing. It is noted on the chart that the client wears glasses, but at the moment is not wearing them. A nurse talks to the client about this.

Filling Out Forms

In doctors' offices, medical centers, nursing homes, and other health care settings, a client's information is documented on charts, forms, and checklists. In these settings, it seems that "if it's not written down, it didn't happen." Even though computers have made this work easier, it is important that all written information is accurate. Health care workers do this by double-checking the information.

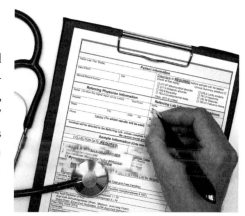

Listening to the Action

Listening for Language

Listen to the conversations between health care workers. What phrases do they use to make sure that the information has been double-checked?

1. _____

2. _____

3. _____

Dialogue

Practicing the Language

A nursing supervisor and nurse at Evergreen Medical Center are discussing the transfer or discharge of several clients. Practice the dialogue with a partner.

Supervisor: Let's review the transfers and discharges for today.

Nurse: O.K. We have the woman with congestive heart failure in Bed 212-B who is going to be transferred to Broadview Nursing Home. Her A.D.L. score for feeding and grooming is high, but she is very dependent in terms of her bathing and toileting.

Supervisor: Right, it's evident that she can't return home in her condition, but I thought that her chart stated that she is going to be released to Parma Lakes Nursing Home, not Broadview. Let's double-check that.

Nurse: Will do. And her roommate, 212-A, who had the heart surgery last week . . . from what the doctor has seen of her recovery, she'll be discharged later today. She's been given instructions on how to take care of her scar area at home.

Supervisor: For the most part, clients understand those instructions, but please mark down that I want to confirm that she understands everything.

Nurse: O.K.

Supervisor: Anyone else?

Nurse: The doctors have concluded that Mr. Gerrity needs to enter hospice. His cancer is in an advanced stage, and he is totally dependent for all his A.D.L.s.

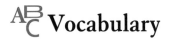 Vocabulary

Activities of Daily Living (ADL) Checklist Terms

Depending on the type of illness or injury a client has, he or she may not be able to do many things without assistance. Health care workers may use a checklist to record how much a client can do. The checklists vary from hospital to hospital, but there are some terms that are very common.

- **Categories:**
  Bathing
  Dressing
  Eating
  Grooming (Hygiene)
  Taking medications
  Managing oral care
  Toileting
  Transferring

- **Scale:**
  Independent
  Needs Assistance
  Dependent
  Does not do (n/a)

Categorizing

Read the key words, and write the appropriate category from this list.

1. bowel movement, involuntary bowel movement, voiding, incontinent, catheter _____

2. correct dosages, correct times _____

3. moving in and out of bed, using cane or walker _____

4. using a toothbrush, cleaning dentures _____

5. feeding self, cutting meat, buttering bread _____

6. selecting clothes, wardrobe, tying shoes _____

7. sponge bath, washing face and hands _____

8. shaving, trimming nails, using deodorant/cologne _____

Scaling

Read the descriptions, and then write the appropriate rating from the scale. The first one has been done for you as an example.

1. Mr. Gould prepares and takes his medications daily. _independent_

2. Mrs. Combs is incontinent while asleep more than once a week. _____

3. Mr. Nehrebecki uses a walker. _____

4. Mrs. Tran needs help pouring her milk and cutting her meat. _____

5. Mr. Coye requires total bathing. _____

6. Mrs. Fett does not wear dentures. _____

7. Mr. Woodworth always dresses neatly and is well-groomed. _____

⇄ Communication Strategy

Double-Checking Information

It is important to make sure that all forms are filled out correctly. Therefore, it is better to double-check important information before writing it instead of making a mistake.

Requests for information to be double-checked
I'd like this to be looked at by another pair of eyes.
I'll just get confirmation on this.
Let's confirm/verify/validate this.
Let's double-check this.

Questions about information after it has been double-checked
Did you use the client's own words?
Has this been double-checked?
Is this confirmed?
Is this correct?
Who else has seen/looked at this?
Who else would know?

Double-Checking Information

Mark an X on the line before information that should be double-checked. Then compare your answers with the class.

1. _____ Incontinent when nurses are in room; bowel/bladder control at night

2. _____ Client walked out of medical center at 3:00 AM. Said he couldn't afford the treatment.

3. _____ Administer 1,000 mgs morphine

4. _____ 901 Main Street, Oakland, CA

5. _____ Arm broken in 5 places

6. _____ Resists efforts of others to feed him

7. _____ Ate 3/4 of her meal

8. _____ The client said she saw a ghost in the room.

Dialogue Completion

New nursing students are learning how to fill out forms. Their supervisor is double-checking what they write. Write an appropriate phrase from the box on page 111 to complete the dialogues.

1. *Student 1:* I think that the doctor said that Mrs. Williams can brush her own teeth.

   Supervisor: _____

2. *Student 2:* Mr. Mason fell down three times in his room today.

   Supervisor: _____

3. *Student 3:* I checked her vitals about four hours ago. I don't remember the exact time.

   Supervisor: _____

4. *Student 4:* I'm writing that the client is coughing continuously.

   Supervisor: _____

Writing Dialogues

Write information about a client that may need to be double-checked. Then, read your sentences to a partner. Your partner will ask for the information to be double-checked. Reverse roles. The first one has been done for you as an example.

1. A: _This client's dinner came with no dessert. She asked us to bring her some cake and ice cream._

   B: "Let's double-check her chart. Maybe she is not allowed to have any dessert."

2. A: _____

   B: _____

3. A: _____

   B: _____

4. A: _____

   B: _____

⇆ Communication Strategy

Drawing Conclusions

When reviewing client information, health care workers draw conclusions about what can be done or must be done. Doctors have the highest authority in the decision-making process, but nurses also need to deal with the recorded information. There are specific phrases to use when drawing a conclusion. If your recommendation for action is strong, you can use a phrase for a stronger conclusion.

Strong Conclusions

Based on this information,
From what we see here,
It's clear that
It's evident that

General Conclusions

For the most part,
It seems that
On the whole,
We have concluded that

Dialogue Practice

Read and practice the dialogues with a partner.

1. *Family Member:* My father looks better today.

   Nurse: Yes, for the most part, his condition is improving. He won't need to be in the hospital much longer.

   Family Member: Wonderful!

2. *Nurse 1:* Miss Baumberger's chart shows that her requests for pain meds are increasing.

   Nurse 2: Yes, it's clear that the dosage she started with when she was admitted is no longer helping her.

3. *Doctor:* Mr. Skokut, your A.D.L. ratings are extremely high. It seems that you are doing well still living alone at 98.

   Client: Well, I just take it one day at a time.

Drawing Conclusions

Write an appropriate conclusion for each of these situations. Then compare your answers with a partner. The first one has been done for you as an example.

1. Karen Scott's A.D.L. checklist shows that she needs help getting out of bed. She cannot ambulate without assistance.

   Based on this information, I recommend that Mrs. Smith's family buy a walker for her to

   use after being discharged.

2. Patrick Simmons' chart shows that he's eaten only about 1/4 of the food served to him at each meal for the last week. He also refuses to drink water between meals.

   _____

   _____.

3. Mr. Snow's dressings have been changed regularly since the accident. His wounds are healing nicely.

   _____

   _____.

4. Mr. Malayang has learned to use several tools to get dressed, even without the use of his left arm.

   _____

   _____.

5. After Miss Jung's infection was treated, the nursing assistants have been checking her mouth regularly for signs of re-infection. They have also taught her how to clean and care for her dentures.

   _____

   _____.

Pronunciation: Primary Sentence Stress

In Unit 3, you learned about basic sentence stress. Most sentences in English have more than one stressed word, but there is always one word that is a little louder, longer, and higher than all of the others. This is called the primary stress. Listen to your instructor read the examples. Which words receive the primary stress?

Charting is usually done by computer

The information must be correct or the doctor won't sign it.

Rule: In many sentences, the primary stress is on the last content word that is stressed in the sentence (the last noun, verb, adjective, or adverb, question word, or negative word). Note that during a conversation, a speaker may give primary stress to any word in the sentence.

Practicing Primary Stress

Read the passages with a partner. Mark each primary stress with a dot.

1. Studying to become a nurse is difficult. There's so much to memorize. It takes a little practice

   to do things right. You need to work at it. It helps to be active in class. Good luck to all of

   you.

2. How are her A.D.L.s? She does well on several of them. She scores high in feeding, dressing,

   and grooming. She just went from a cane to a walker. She needs it.

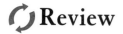 Review

Dialogue Review

Review the dialogue on page 109. As you read, follow the directions. Then compare your answers with a partner.

- Underline the **A.D.L. Checklist** terms.
- Circle the ways to **Double-Check Information**.
- Box the **Drawing Conclusions** phrases.

Role Plays: Filling Out Forms

Work with a partner. Read each situation, and develop a dialogue to perform for the class.

1. A nurse starts to write on a chart that a client has trouble breathing. Her supervisor asks if the information has been double-checked.

2. A nurse and a client are talking about how many of the family members visit each day. The nurse draws a conclusion about the client and the family members.

3. Two nurses discuss a client who has suffered a stroke. They discuss the client's scores in the bathing, dressing, toileting, and grooming categories.

4. A doctor and a supervisor discuss a client who seems ready to be discharged but who may need some care at home.

5. A nursing student checks the box for "client refuses to eat" on a checklist. A nurse thinks that client is eating. They discuss the issue.

6. A supervisor and a nurse are discussing a client who has been improving. The supervisor draws a conclusion about the client.

7. A home health care worker interviews an elderly woman in her home. She asks her about items on the A.D.L. checklist.

End-of-Unit Discussion

Sharing

Discuss the questions with a small group.

1. Why are confirmation checks important to use?

2. Give some examples of abbreviations that are very easy to remember and some that are very difficult to remember.

3. Since charting is so important, are you worried that you will spend more time charting than actually taking care of clients? Do you think that this problem will improve or get worse?

4. Which of the A.D.L.s do elderly people have trouble with first? Which of the A.D.L.s are still relatively easy for elderly people?

Culture Point: Fate

Read this story. Discuss in small groups and as a class.

————

Yolanda was talking to an Environmental Services worker, Bandhi, in the break room. Bandhi told Yolanda what happened earlier that day . . .

Bandhi: My supervisor told me that next year he'll recommend that I can start training to become a supervisor myself. He said that it's clear that I will eventually manage a department here, and then maybe even secure a job overseeing Environmental Services at another hospital.

Yolanda: Good for you!

Bandhi: But how can he say that!?

————

Why is Bandhi surprised?

UNIT 7: Exchanging Information during Shift Changes

Shift change is one of the most important times to have clear communication. It is the time between shifts when information is exchanged about each client. These updates need to be clearly understood.

Reporting Live Client Handovers

Some facilities report shift information live. That is, the head nurse gives the information face to face. Sometimes the entire health care staff needs to hear this report. There may be times when some of the details are not completely clear. Since this report is live, there is a chance to clarify information with the speaker. It is also good to summarize or repeat or review the main points of the report in other words. Summarizing is an important skill to use in conversations too.

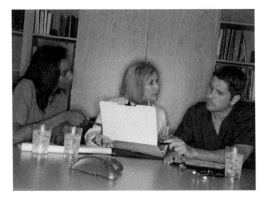

Listening to the Action

 ### Listening for Language

Listen to the conversations between colleagues in health care setting. What phrases do the second speakers use to summarize?

1. _____

2. _____

3. _____

⇅ Dialogue

Practicing the Language

The off-going charge nurse is reporting to the on-coming nurses. Practice the dialogue with a partner.

Charge Nurse: Hello, everybody. Let's go over the details from the last 12 hours. The appendectomy in 403 needs to be discharged March 5th, so we need to do the final check-up tomorrow. Recovery is going well. Fluid intake normal and all output regular.

Nurse: Sorry, the appendectomy in 403 needs to be discharged when?

Charge Nurse: March 5th, the day after tomorrow.

Nurse: Thank you.

Charge Nurse: We have a new admit in 414. Scott Whitman, 44, male. Diagnosed with H1N1. Dr. Abdul's admit. Client has a history of respiratory issues. Currently short of breath and running a temp of 104°. Tylenol given at 2:00 PM. All vitals normal besides an elevated blood pressure.

Nurse: It sounds like we need to attend to him first.

Charge Nurse: Yes. And please record vital signs again, instruct Mr. Whitman on the oxygen mask, and inform him why he needs to be in respiratory isolation.

Nurse: Got it.

ABC Vocabulary

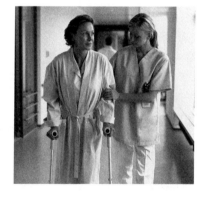

Work Duties

There are many different duties to perform in medical facilities. Health care workers should be familiar with these duties when they listen during a shift change. Some certified nursing assistant (CNA) and registered nurse (RN) duties are listed.

CNA

- **do/make** rounds
- **drop off** supper trays
- **get** hallway assignment
- **get** reports
- **pass out** linens
- **record** list of vitals
- **reposition** the client
- **toilet** the client
- **transfer** residents

RN

- **assess** the client
- **call** doctors to report assessments
- **check** crash cart
- **check** meds
- **do** rounds with doctors
- **have** a unit meeting
- **inform** the client's family
- **instruct** the client
- **regroup** with staff

Sentence Completion

Complete the sentences with the correct word from the list on page 119.

1. It's after the lunch break. We should _____ with staff now.

2. First I will _____ of vitals, O.K.?

3. Let's get Sandra to _____ the linens this time

4. You need to _____ Mr. Conley from the I.C.U. at noon.

5. Please _____ rounds with Dr. Pageman in ten minutes.

Sentence Writing

Choose five duties from the list on page 119. Write a sentence showing you understand the meaning of the word or phrase. The first one has been done for you as an example.

1. *I need to transfer Ms. Hoff from Radiology to his room at 5:00 PM.*

2. _____

3. _____

4. _____

5. _____

6. _____

⇄ Communication Strategy

Clarification Requests

Sometimes you do not understand everything you hear or hear everything people say. You need to understand the important details of a message to make communcation successful. A good way to do this is to repeat the request and use a question word. You can use a question word in place of the word you did not hear or understand.

Formal

    I'm sorry. You need what?
    Pardon me. It's where?
    Excuse me. Who will be coming?

Less Formal

    Sorry. Help you with what?
    Sorry. The client went where?
    Sorry. Who needs assistance?

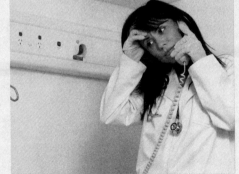

Dialogue Practice

Read and practice the dialogues with a partner.

1. *Nurse:*   I need a vitals sheet right now.

   Nursing Assistant: Excuse me. You need a what?

   Nurse: I need a vitals sheet.

2. *Client:*   Can you help me with my I.V.

   Nurse: I'm sorry. Help you with what?

   Client: My I.V., my I.V. It's coming out!

3. *Head Nurse:*   Mr. Lamperts needs assistance in 314-B.

   Nurse: Pardon me. Who needs assistance?

   Head Nurse: Mr. Lamperts. He needs to eliminate.

Dialogue Completion

Complete the questions and statements in the first column with a word or phrase that you might hear in a medical setting. Then complete the questions in the second column with the correct *wh-* question word. The first one has been done for you as an example.

1. "Can I have a drink of ____water____?"   I'm sorry. A drink of ____what____?

2. "Can I have a little _____?"   Pardon me. Have a little _____?

3. "I need to go to _____!"   Sorry. You need to go _____?

4. "My _____ is going to visit me."   Excuse me. _____ is coming to visit you?

5. "Nurse! I would really love _____." Sorry. You would really love _____?

6. "Please come to station 5 at _____." Excuse me. Come to station 5 _____?

Dialogue Practice

Read and practice the dialogues with a partner. Reverse roles.

⇆ Communication Strategy

Summarizing

It's important that you make the person that you are speaking with know that you are listening, that you understand, and that you are interested. To do this, you can repeat the important parts in your own words. This is called a summary. If your summary is incorrect, the other person can help correct the information. This skill takes practice, but there are several phrases you can use to begin your summaries.

In other words

In summary

It sounds like

To sum up

What you're saying is (that)

You mean

Dialogue Practice

Read and practice the dialogues with a partner.

1. *Head Nurse:*   You will need an oral or auxiliary thermometer to check temperature, a watch to check respiratory and pulse rates, and a stethoscope and blood pressure cuff to check blood pressure.

   Nurse: In other words, prepare the materials to check vitals.

2. *Nursing Assistant 1:* I think I have always been on time, work very hard, and am always extra friendly to clients.

   Nursing Assistant 2: You mean you want a promotion?

3. *Doctor:*   The client gets no food or water for 12 hours. Make sure he has eliminated as much as possible. I need all lab tests and results to me before we operate.

   Nurse: It sounds like the client will have a major procedure.

Dialogue Completion

Complete the dialogues with a summary. Begin your summary with a phrase from the box on page 122.

1. *A:* I have a headache, my chest hurts, and I feel hot.

   B: _____.

2. *A.* One nurse said, "So long, lady" in Tagalog to another nurse. A client started to panic because *"Sige na 'day"* was heard as *"She's gonna die!"*

   B: _____.

3. *A:* Yesterday I got in a car accident, my boyfriend broke up with me, and one of my clients died.

   B: _____.

4. *A:* Mr. Dugan in 515-A talked about his childhood, his job, his family, his hobbies, and his views on politics. I listened to him as long as I could. Be careful in there!

   B: _____.

Discussion

Talk about these topics with a partner. Take turns summarizing each other's story.

1. Why you are working / want to work in the health care field

2. A problem you have

3. The rules of your favorite sport or game

4. Your favorite person

5. The last movie you saw

Pronunciation: Moving the Primary Stress

Unit 6 talks about the primary stress being on the last content word (noun, verb, adjective, adverb) in the sentence. However, it is possible to move the primary stress to any word in the sentence. The speaker decides where to put the stress depending on the situation. Listen to your instructor read the two sentences. Notice the change in the primary stress.

Where is that client's chart?

Where is that client's chart?

I speak English. →   not other people

I speak English. →   not read it

I speak English. →   not another language.

<u>Rule</u>: The meaning of a sentence changes if the primary stress is moved. Primary stress can even be on a word that isn't normally stressed (a pronoun, possessive adjective, etc.).

Listening

Listen to your instructor read the sentences. Mark the stressed words.

1. a. How long do we set the timer?   b. How long do we set the timer?

2. a. Which bandage should I use?   b. Which bandage should I use?

3. a. When will the relatives come?   b. When will the relatives come?

4. a. Where do I record the vitals?   b. Where do I record the vitals?

5. a. Why did he get a second meal?   b. Why did he get a second meal?

6. a. Who needs to be repositioned?   b. Who needs to be repositioned?

Listening for Primary Stress

Listen to your instructor read one of the sentences from each set. Mark the sentence you hear based on the location of the primary stress.

1. ___ a. Anne is switching to Community General next **month.** (not any other time)

   ___ b. Anne is switching to Community General **next** month. (not a different month)

   ___ c. Anne is switching to **Community General** next month. (not another hospital)

   ___ d. **Anne** is switching to Community General next month. (not anyone else)

2. ___ a. When did you finish your **shift?** (not any other thing that you finished)

   ___ b. When did you **finish** your shift? (not start it)

   ___ c. When did **you** finish your shift? (not anyone else)

   ___ d. **When** did you finish your shift? (what time exactly)

3. ___ a. Show the son of the client in Room 902 how to feed her the **soup.** (what?)

   ___ b. Show the son of the client in Room 902 **how** to feed her the soup. (how?)

   ___ c. Show the son of the client in **Room 902** how to feed her the soup. (where?)

   ___ d. Show **the son** of the client in Room 902 how to feed her the soup. (who?)

Writing Sentences

Write four sentences. Read them with a partner, and practice stressing different words to give the sentence different meanings each time.

1. _____.

2. _____.

3. _____.

4. _____.

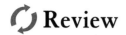 # Review

Dialogue Review

Review the dialogue on page 119. As you read, follow the directions. Then compare your answers with a partner.

- Underline the **Work Duty** terms.
- Circle the **Clarification Request**.
- Box the **Summarizing** phrase.

Role Plays: Live Handovers

Work with a partner. Read each situation, and develop a dialogue to perform for the class.

1. A charge nurse states, "Bob Bolen, Jr., kidney stones, was just admitted to Room 314." A nurse asks for clarification of the room number.

2. A charge nurse tells a nurse, "Toilet the client in Room 421-B, then reposition the client on his side, and call his doctor to report your assessments." The nurse summarizes these instructions.

3. A charge nurse states, "Yoko Nakane, a client we have all grown to love, will be discharged tomorrow." A nurse asks for a summary of Yoko's condition, and the charge nurse responds.

4. A charge nurse states, "Diane Christine, Room 410, has been transferred to another unit." A nurse asks for clarification of the unit.

5. A CNA asks if she can learn to check meds. Her supervisor explains that there are many things that a CNA is not allowed to do.

6. A supervisor at a skilled nursing facility tells a nurse, "Make rounds with the CNA, check the crash cart, help transfer the residents to the dining area, and then check the meds please." The nurse summarizes these instructions.

7. A charge nurse states, "The client in bed 701-A, Mr. Chen, has had a dozen visitors during this last shift. The visits are expected to continue." A nurse summarizes the situation.

Giving Shift Reports

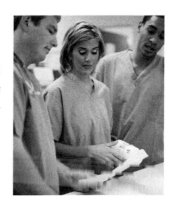

Vital information reports are given during shift changes. It is essential to have your listening skills ready for this. You may not have a chance to ask questions to clarify. You should focus on the order of the information and action words. Good note-taking skills are also necessary.

Listening to the Action

Listening for Language

Listen to the health care workers giving instructions. What work duties do they give?

1. _____

2. _____

3. _____

Dialogue

Practicing the Language

A group of nurses is listening to a shift report during a shift change. Practice the dialogue in groups of three.

Charge Nurse:	Hello, night shift. Welcome to the craziness. Since this report has a lot of information, I will go over my instructions clearly. First. . . .
Nurse (to other nurse):	O.K., let's take notes now.
Charge Nurse:	The CNAs need to check the cath bags. Second, they need to change the wet pads, if necessary. Third, please conduct skin assessments. Finally, give a bed bath to all six clients on this floor. I hope you got that.
CNA:	Did she say conduct skin assessments?
Nurse 2:	Yes, I think she did.
Charge Nurse:	O.K. Next, I will talk about preparations for Derek Wilson's heart surgery.

Vocabulary

More Work Duties

Nursing positions carry a list of responsibilities. More CNA and RN duties are listed.

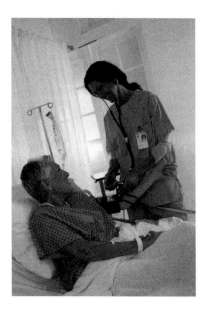

- **CNA**
  change wet pads
  check cath bags
  check reports
  complete documentation
  conduct skin assessments
  do paperwork
  give bed baths
  give unmedicated creams
  lotion the client
  take vitals

- **RN**
  call the pharmacy
  change dressings
  draw labs
  give discharge orders
  start an IV
  stock supplies
  strip discharge beds
  teach clients a procedure
  turn surgical clients
  write telephone and standing orders

Sentence Completion

Complete the sentences with the correct word from the lists.

1. I need to _____ the dressing on Room 414's neck wound.

2. We should never forget to _____ the report before beginning a shift.

3. After you _____ the discharge beds, can you _____ an I.V. in Room 507.

4. Did someone _____ the surgical clients yet?

5. Well, since it's slow, why don't I _____ the supplies?

Charades

Work with a small group. Take turns acting out words from the lists on page 128. Your group members will guess the word.

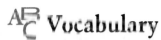 Vocabulary

Frequency of Duties

Sometimes you need to describe how often you perform certain actions. Some of those words are used before the main verb. Each has its own meaning. Read the list and examples.

always	I **always** strip discharge beds. (100%)
usually	I **usually** help my co-workers. (80%)
sometimes	I **sometimes** give a bed bath. (50%)
rarely	I **rarely** come in late. (20%)
never	I **never** forget my reports. (0%)

Other phrases to describe frequency are placed at the end of the sentence.

every month	I check my time sheet **every month**.
every week	I go to a floor meeting **every week**.
every day	I use the equipment **every day**.
every hour	I organize my station **every hour**.

Dialogue Completion

Write answers to the questions. Then, ask your partner the questions. Reverse roles.

1. *A:* How often do you organize your work station?

   B: I organize my work station _____.

2. *A:* How often do you come in late?

   B: I _____ come in late.

3. *A:* How often do you strip discharge beds?

   B: I strip discharge beds _____.

4. *A:* How often do you stock supplies?

   B: I stock supplies _____.

Discussion

Describe what you do at work and how often you do it.

⇆ Communication Strategy

Listening to Instructions

Instructions are everywhere. You must listen to your instructions from your parents, your instructors, and your supervisor. You need to learn how to listen to instructions to help you learn new things. Listening actively and taking notes will help.

Sentence Completion

Listen to these instructions from a supervisor or a client (your teacher). Complete the statements with the words that you hear.

1. Please _____ the box and _____ it with the carton.

2. I need you to _____ the lights in the lab.

3. Can you _____ a client lift? I want you to _____ Jose Diaz.

4. Please _____ the plastic wrap from the applicator and _____ it on the sheet.

5. I want you to _____ my TV.

6. Can you _____ the trash and wipe the tables?

7. Please _____ Room 606's bathroom and _____ the beds.

8. I need you to help me _____ the heart-rate machine, please.

Active Listening

Listen to the instructions as your teacher reads them. Number the sentences in the order you hear them.

1. **Beginning an Assessment or Procedure**

    _____ Explain the procedure

    _____ Greet the client

    _____ Ask client about his or her condition

    _____ Begin the procedure

    _____ Introduce yourself

    _____ Confirm identity of client

2. **Dealing with Client Problems**

    _____ Solve the problem.

    _____ Listen to the client.

    _____ Say thank you.

    _____ Apologize.

⇆ Communication Strategy

Telling a Story

Life is full of stories. Everyone grows up with stories, and everyone has many personal stories. You also hear stories from clients and from co-workers. They can be funny stories, sad stories, exciting stories, or work stories. Stories are always told in the past, so they need past tense verbs. Stories also have an order and the order is indicated by using sequential words.

Sequential Words

One time	First
Then	Next
After that	Finally

Regular Past Tense Verbs
walked
joined
painted

Irregular Past Tense Verbs
drank
caught
ran

Writing Instructions

Write your own step by step instructions. Use words such as *first, then,* or *finally* to connect the steps. Read your instructions to a partner. One has been done for you as an example.

How to make a hamburger:
First, barbeque the ground beef.
Then, put the meat on a bun.
Next, put lettuce and tomato on it.
Then, add ketchup and mustard.
Finally, put another bun on the top.

Title: _____

First, _____

Then, _____

Next, _____

Then, _____

Finally, _____

Dialogue Practice

Underline the sequence words. Then read and practice the story with a partner.

Funny Story in the ED

One time a family ran into the ED with their baby. At first we were a little worried. Then, we asked what had happened. Next, they explained that the baby hadn't smiled for one hour! They said the baby always smiles. Finally, we tried to hold back the laughter and told them everything was O.K.

Listening to a Story

Listen to a student tell a funny or interesting story. Then answer the questions.

1. What happened first? _____

2. What happened last? _____

3. What verbs were used?

   _____, _____, _____

   _____, _____, _____

   _____, _____, _____

Story Order

Put the story in order. Write 1 by the first thing that happened and 6 for the last thing that happened. Fill in the events in between. Then compare your answers with a partner.

_____ Finally, he stabilized.

_____ Then, I called for help

_____ First, he started to have a reaction.

_____ Next, I saw his eyes roll back into his head.

_____ One time I saw a client come back from surgery.

_____ The doctor was close by, so we were lucky.

Telling a Story

Think of a story about one of the topics. Write it on the lines, and then read it to the class.

1. A story from my childhood

2. My first day on the job

3. A funny story

4. A hospital story

One time _____

First, _____

Then, _____

Next, _____

Then, _____

Finally, _____

Pronunciation: Past Tense Endings

When we talk about things that happened in the past, regular verbs end with an *-ed*.

"I pick**ed** up the phone, dial**ed** the number, and wait**ed** for someone to answer."

Rule: The way that the *-ed* is pronounced depends on the last sound in the word.

Type A: Short ending: Usually, the *-ed* at the end of a past tense verb does not add an extra syllable.
Listen and repeat the examples.

live → live**d**	help → help**ed**
work → work**ed**	bandage → bandag**ed**
learn → learn**ed**	finish → finish**ed**
play → play**ed**	watch → watch**ed**
smile → smil**ed**	drop → dropp**ed**
clean → clean**ed**	listen → listen**ed**

Type B: Long ending: When the last sound in the verb is *t* or *d*, we add an extra syllable.
Listen and repeat the examples.

want → want**ed**	faint → faint**ed**
need → need**ed**	complete → complet**ed**
wait → wait**ed**	decide → decid**ed**
start → start**ed**	conduct → conduct**ed**
end → end**ed**	hand → hand**ed**

Past Tense Verbs

Write the past tense of the verbs. Then practice the pronunciation with a partner.

1. move _____
2. hurry _____
3. stay _____
4. slip _____
5. walk _____

6. wash _____
7. rub _____
8. pick _____
9. care _____
10. call _____

Recognizing Past Tense Verbs

Read the sentences. Circle the verbs that have a past tense /d/ sound.

1. During her shift, Nurse Ann cared for six clients in the pediatric ward.

2. She checked on them each hour.

3. She turned their position every hour.

4. She called the doctor when they were in pain.

5. She listened to their worries and soothed them.

Extra Syllable Past Tense Verbs

Write the past tense of the verbs. Then practice the pronunciation with a partner.

1. invite	_____	6. count	_____
2. visit	_____	7. operate	_____
3. attend	_____	8. correct	_____
4. add	_____	9. succeed	_____
5. subtract	_____	10. record	_____

Recognizing Extra Syllable Past Tense Verbs

Read the sentences. Circle the verbs that have the extra syllable after the past tense -ed ending is added.

1. Everyone attended the staff meeting at the beginning of the shift.

2. Our supervisor counted us, and we were all there.

3. She added a new step to the electronic charting procedure.

4. She corrected some information from the last meeting.

5. And, she invited us to the holiday party.

Using Past Tense Verbs

Choose a word or phrase from each column, and include all three in a sentences. Write eight sentences. Then practice them with a partner.

Subject	Verb	Object
Hospital staff members	mopped	some beds
The kitchen workers	stripped	the toilets
The nurse's aides	answered	the dishwasher
Environmental services workers	cooked	the floor
Home health care workers	disinfected	the towels
	folded	the phone
	admitted	the meals
	loaded	clients

1. _____

2. _____

3. _____

4. _____

5. _____

6. _____

7. _____

8. _____

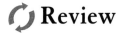 # Review

Dialogue Review

Review the dialogue on page 127. As you read, follow the directions. Then compare your answers with a partner.

- Underline the **Work Duty** terms.
- Circle the **Verbs in Instructions**.
- Box the **Sequential Words**.

Role Plays: Shift Reports

Work with a partner. Read each situation, and develop a dialogue to perform for the class.

1. Two nurses are listening to a shift report. They are confused about whether they heard *intolerance* or *incontinence*. They decide to ask the supervisor.

2. At the end of a shift, two nurses talk about what they did during their shift.

3. Two nurses hear at a shift change that a client that they liked a lot died overnight. Their reaction is emotional. They talk about wishing that they could have been there the night before.

4. A client asks a CNA to do various tasks. The CNA lets the client know which work duties can be done.

5. Two nurses are giving a report to the next shift. They are talking about Mr. Wences in 401-B. One reports on the I.V. bag she hung. The other reports that his K this morning was 3.2 and the K needs to be repeated at 8:00 PM.

6. A CNA wants the experience of giving a discharge order. An RN explains to a CNA why only RNs can give discharge orders.

7. Two nursing students compare the work duties that they always do and the work duties that they never do.

End-of-Unit Discussion

Sharing

Discuss the questions with a small group.

1. Which of the work duties in this unit are easiest or will be easiest for you? Which are or will be the most difficult?

2. What is your ideal shift in terms of start time and end time? Do you think that you would be happy working in the middle of the night?

3. A nurse or CNA is sometimes tired at the end of a shift. How can you keep your nursing skills sharp at the end of a shift?

4. When is it necessary to tell a story about a client (of course, not using that client's name)? Give an example.

Culture Point: Finishing Work on Time

Read this story. Discuss in small groups and as a class.

A new CNA, Rachel, was having trouble finishing her tasks by the end of her shift. Debra, a nurse supervisor, offered to help. When Rachel said that she didn't need help, Debra said, "Don't be crazy. Let me help you. Your shift is over and you need to leave."

Rachel started shaking and quickly left the area.

Why was Rachel upset?

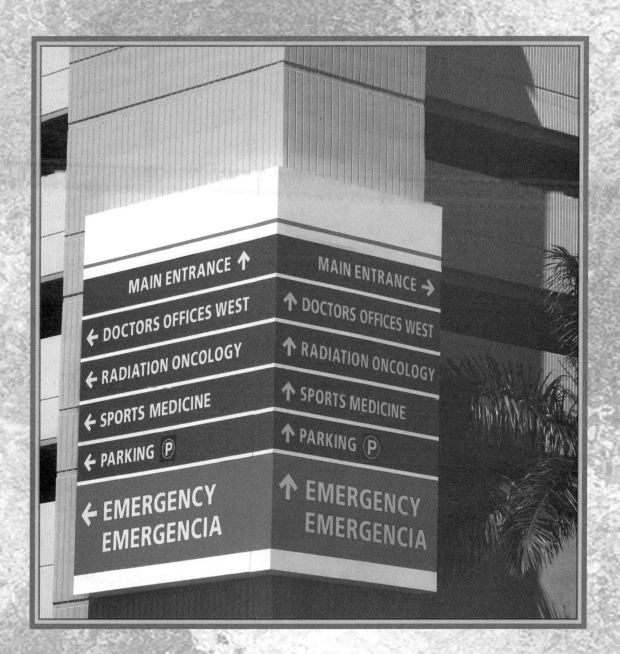

PART 4

Around the Facility

UNIT 8: Knowing Facility Locations

No two medical facilities (hospitals, clinics, medical offices) are exactly alike. Some rooms, such as waiting rooms or restrooms can be found in all medical facilities, but there are dozens of specific locations that may be in one facility and not another. It is important to know the floor plan for the facility where you work.

Learning Locations

Even though you may only need to work in the same few rooms each day for your particular job, a large medical center consists of many specialized areas. A few areas of a hospital resemble a typical office building, but most locations are highly specialized. It is important for all health care workers to be familiar with all the locations in a medical center and to know what happens in those locations. It is a good idea to be able to compare facilities.

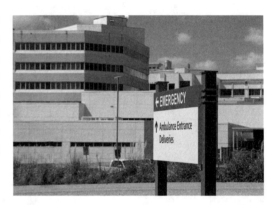

Listening to the Action

Listening for Language

Listen to the conversations between health care workers. What specific locations are they comparing?

1. _____

2. _____

3. _____

⇅ Dialogue

Practicing the Language

A teenager receives permission from a hospital to spend one day with her aunt, who is an RN in the oncology ward. She wants to be a nursing student when she goes to college. They are talking as they walk through the hallways. Practice the dialogue with a partner.

Teenager: Hey, thanks for letting me "shadow" you today, Aunt Carrie.

Nurse: No problem, Lani. I hope that you learn a lot. Feel free to ask a lot of questions.

Teenager: O.K. What's the busiest place in a hospital?

Nurse: Well, all parts of a hospital can be busy, but I'd say that the ED is usually busier than other places.

Teenager: Did you ever work in the ED?

Nurse: Yes, at one time I did, but I prefer working in the oncology ward now.

Teenager: Why?

Nurse: Well, Lani, when most people hear the word *cancer,* they are afraid. I like to make them less afraid, especially because there is so much advanced technology in hospitals now.

Teenager: Oh, look. Here's a sign that says Pediatrics. What happens there?

Nurse: Oh, that's the area of the hospital where doctors and nurses take care of children.

Teenager: Children? Great! I think I've decided on what kind of nurse I want to be. A children's nurse!

Nurse: You mean a pediatric nurse. Yes, that *is* great!

ᴬᴮC Vocabulary

Locations within a Medical Facility

Although some locations in a medical facility (classroom, restroom) are also in other types of buildings, others (surgery, radiology) are very specific to a hospital. Some of these locations in a medical center are named for people who have contributed greatly to the success of the facility either with their time, expertise, or donation. One example is the *Shaker Family Eye Clinic.*

- **General**

auditorium	elevators	recovery room	unit
classroom	entrance	reception area	waiting room
client's room	hallway	restroom	ward
clinic	laboratory	staff room	wing
conference room	lobby	stairs	
department	office	supply room	

- **Specific**

cafeteria/coffee shop	Emergency	Medical Records	pharmacy
Cardiovascular	Department	Office	Physical Therapy
Surgery	gift shop	Oncology	Radiology (X-Ray)
chapel/meditation	Labor and	Outpatient Center	Surgery
room	Delivery	Pediatrics	Trauma

Categorizing

List medical center locations that fit into each category. There may be more than three answers for each category.

1. Locations that are similar in meaning to *ward*

   a. _____

   b. _____

   c. _____

2. Locations where doctors operate on clients

   a. _____

   b. _____

   c. _____

3. Locations where teaching and learning occur

   a. _____

   b. _____

   c. _____

4. Locations where money is used

   a. _____

   b. _____

   c. _____

5. Locations that could be named after someone

   a. _____

   b. _____

   c. _____

Locations

Label each location according to who goes there. If it is a place nurses or other health care workers usually go, write N on the line. If it is a place where visitors usually go, write V on the line. If it is a place where both health care workers and visitors usually go, write B for both.

1. chapel _____

2. Labor and Delivery _____

3. Radiology _____

4. restroom _____

5. gift shop _____

6. supply room _____

7. Surgery _____

8. waiting room _____

9. pharmacy _____

10. cafeteria _____

⇆ Communication Strategy

Describing the Functions of Locations

Newly hired health care workers might need to ask about a part of a hospital that they aren't familiar with. More commonly, clients or family members might ask about the function of locations in the hospital. You need to be familiar with these questions so you can answer them.

What do people do in a _____ ?

What's the function of a _____ ?

What happens in a _____ ?

Who works in a _____ ?

Is a _____ where a doctor/client _____ ?

Who/Which type of client needs to go to a _____ ?

Is the _____ here like a _____ in a different hospital?

Do all hospitals have a _____ ?

Dialogue Completion

Complete the dialogues, and then practice them with a partner.

1. *Client:*   Is a _____ where a client goes for _____?
   Nurse: Yes, x-rays are taken there.

2. *Relative:*   Is the Meditation Garden here like a _____ in a different hospital?
   Nurse: Yes, it's like an outdoor chapel.

3. *New Nurse:* Do all hospitals have a _____?
   Nurse: No, only the biggest hospitals have one.

Writing Responses

Answer the questions in your own words.

1. What is the function of a recovery room?

   _____.

2. What happens in a medical records room?

   _____.

3. Who works in an oncology center?

   _____.

⇆ Communication Strategy

Making Comparisons

Some locations within a medical center are the same wherever you go. Others are very different. It's possible to make comparisons between locations in medical centers using specific words and phrases.

advanced technology/state of the art technology/cutting-edge technology

better equipped than/less well-equipped than

busier than/slower than

different/similar

identical

larger than/smaller than

more centrally located

more spacious than/less spacious than

newer than or older than

safer than/more hazardous than

slightly different/somewhat different

the same

versus

Sentence Completion

Complete the sentences with an appropriate phrase from the box.

1. The Cleveland Clinic was established in 1921, which means that it's _____ more modern hospitals.

2. The client rooms in the East Wing and the West Wing are _____.

3. The newest hospitals have _____ technology.

4. A private client room is _____ than a shared client room.

5. Instead of putting the A.T.M. machines only in the cafeterias, hospitals are making sure that A.T.M.s are _____.

6. Older floor plans are generally less spacious and thus _____. Accidents can happen more often with less room to move around.

Making Comparisons

Use the floor plan to write comparisons between these locations on the floor plan and a facility you are familiar with.

1. cafeteria: _____.

2. lobby: _____.

3. gift shop: _____.

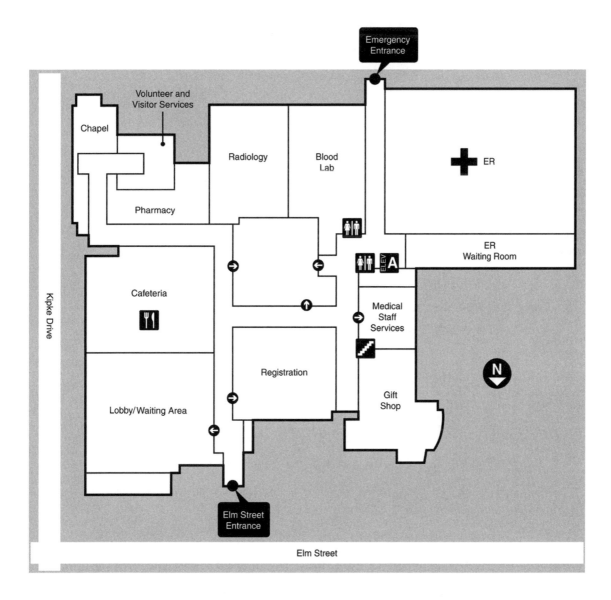

Pronunciation: Compound Nouns

A compound noun is one word made from two separate words. Listen to your instructor read the examples. Which syllable is stressed?

toothpaste   headache

<u>Rule</u>: The first word in a compound noun carries more stress than the second.

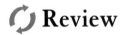 ## Compound Nouns

Mark the stress on the compound nouns and then practice the pronunciation with a partner.

1. wheelchair	5. courtyard	9. washcloth
2. drugstore	6. bedpan	10. glassware
3. notebook	7. roommate	11. pillowcase
4. audiometer	8. underwear	12. restroom

Review

Dialogue Review

Review the dialogue on page 141. As you read, follow the directions. Then compare you answers with a partner.

- Underline the **Locations within a Medical Facility**.
- Circle the phrase that **Describes a Function of a Location**.
- Box the **Comparison Words**.

Role Plays: Locations

Work with a partner. Read each situation, and develop a dialogue to perform for the class.

1. Two nursing students compare their classroom to another classroom they know.

2. A client from another culture asks a nurse what an outpatient lab is used for.

3. A family member gets lost and enters a staff room. An environmental services worker gives directions to help the person get back into a public area.

4. Two nurses discuss the advantages a newer hospital may have over an older hospital.

5. A new nurse asks her supervisor if the client rooms in the medical center are similar to the ones in other hospitals.

6. A client's family member asks a nurse what the difference is between a staff room and a waiting room.

7. An elderly client requests a new washcloth, pillowcase, and underwear from a nursing assistant.

Getting around the Facility

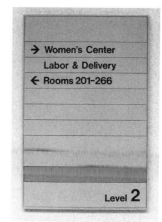

Medical facilities vary in size. Even if a facility is small, the first time a new employee or a visitor enters, that person will need to find various locations (waiting areas, client rooms, restrooms, the cafeteria, the gift shop, the pharmacy, or the chapel). Signs are helpful, but many people ask for directions anyway. It is important to give clear and complete directions using the correct prepositions.

Listening to the Action

Listening for Language

Listen to the conversations between health care workers and visitors. What prepositions do the health care workers use to give directions?

1. _____

2. _____

3. _____

⇅ Dialogue

Practicing the Language

During a busy shift, a staff member at the reception desk in the lobby of a large hospital directs many visitors to where they need to go. Practice the dialogue in groups of five.

Visitor 1:	Can you tell me where the children's ward is?
Staff Member:	It's on the 5th floor. Turn right as you get out of the elevator, and you'll see it right in front of you. It's a piece of cake. You can't miss it.
Visitor 1:	Thanks.
Staff Member:	You're welcome.
Staff Member (to Visitor 2):	Good morning. May I help you?
Visitor 2:	Yes, I got a call that my son has been taken to emergency. Where do I go?
Staff Member:	Go down this hall [points] until it ends. The ED waiting room is on the left. There's a large sign.
Visitor 2:	O.K.
Visitor 3:	Excuse me. Can you point me in the direction of the patient rooms?
Staff Member:	There are many floors with client rooms. What kind of illness does the client have?
Visitor 3:	Illness? Oh, no. She just had a baby!

The sign shown reads:

→ Women's Center
Labor & Delivery
← Rooms 201-266

Level 2

Staff Member:	Oh, Maternity is on the 3rd floor in the West Wing. Take this elevator up. Turn left when you get off, and then follow the signs that say West Wing. You'll see the nurses' station there, and you can ask for the room number.
Visitor 3:	Thanks for your help.
Staff Member:	No problem.
Visitor 4:	I'm lost! I don't know which way to turn. I parked in the parking garage, but now I don't know how to get back there.
Staff Member:	Oh, don't worry. This place is big. Here's a map. Here's where we are, and here's the parking garage. Have a nice day.

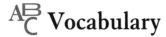 Vocabulary

Prepositions and Adverbs of Place

We use prepositions and adverbs of place to talk about locations.

- **Prepositions:** *on, at, in, by, near, next to, behind, between, down*
  The Radiology Lab is on the third floor.

- **Adverbs of place:** *here, there, over there*
  The supply closet is here.

Sentence Completion

Complete the sentences with the correct preposition.

1. The nurses are _____ their station.

2. The medical offices are _____ the West Wing.

3. The Emergency Department is _____ the back entrance of the hospital.

4. The Nursery? It's _____ the delivery room.

5. The main lobby is _____ the North Wing and the South Wing.

6. The restrooms are _____. Can you see them?

7. The coffee shop is _____, around the corner.

Reading a Floor Plan

Look at the hospital floor plan on page 145. Complete the sentences with the correct preposition.

1. Radiology is _____ the blood labs.

2. The ER is _____ the restroom.

3. The lobby is _____ the Elm Street entrance.

4. The cafeteria is _____ the lobby.

5. There is one elevator on this floor. It's _____ the ER waiting room.

⇆ Communication Strategy

Asking for and Giving Directions

Hospitals, health centers, and clinics are big places. It is important to be able to ask for and give directions.

Direction Words

Go down the hall.	Go straight ahead.
Go down the stairs.	Go up the stairs.
Go left.	Take the elevator down.
Go past the exit.	Take the elevator up.
Go right.	Turn left.
Go straight.	Turn right.

It's on the left.
It's on the right.
It's right in front of you.

Idioms

I don't know which way to turn.
It's a piece of cake.
You can't miss it.

Hospital Visitor: Where is the nurses station for the Oncology Unit?

You: Oncology? It's **on** the third floor. From the elevators, **turn left. Go past** the restrooms. It's **on the right.**

Giving Directions

Role play giving directions from one place in the school to another. Use your hands to gesture as you give directions.

Using Direction Words

Look at the hospital floor plan on page 145. Take turns asking for directions and giving directions for the places,

1. from the cafeteria to the restrooms

2. from the cafeteria to the gift shop

3. from the lobby to the chapel

4. from registration to the blood lab

5. from the lobby to the ED waiting room

⇆ Communication Strategy

Giving Longer or More Complex Directions

It is easy to have a communication breakdown when giving directions. Sometimes the location is so far away that the directions are very long and complicated. Sometimes the person who asks for directions is elderly and may not hear well or may be confused. In these cases, it might be better to get a map, draw a map, or even take the visitor to the location. For longer and more complex directions, use these phrases to help.

First, say:
>   It's complicated.
>   It's far.
>   It's not easy to find.

Then say:
>   I'll get someone to show you. Just a minute.
>   I'm going that way. I'll take you there.
>   I'll show you. Come with me.
>   Let me draw it for you.
>   Let me draw you a map.
>   Let me get you a hospital map/floor plan.
>   Let me mark that for you on a map.
>   The pharmacy is here. (Point to the floor plan or mark the floor plan.)

Sentence Completion

Fill in the blanks with an appropriate word or phrase from the box on page 150.

1. *Visitor:*   Where is the prenatal classroom?

   Hospital Worker: It's a little far. I'll _____ you there.

2. *Visitor:*   I need to find the Nutrition Counseling room.

   Hospital Worker: Let me _____ you a map and _____ it for you.

3. *Visitor:*   I've been told to take the F Elevator. Where is that?

   Hospital Worker: Follow me. I'll _____ you.

Pronunciation: Two-Word Nouns

There are many two-word nouns in English. Listen to your instructor read the examples. Which word is stressed?

snack bar   laundry room

Rule: The first word in a two-word noun carries more stress than the second word.

Two-Word Nouns

Mark the stress on these two-word nouns, and then practice the pronunciation by using the words in a sentence with a partner.

1. Emergency Department	5. Maternity Ward	9. physician's entrance
2. Radiology Lab	6. medical center	10. Children's Ward
3. East Wing	7. x-ray machine	11. family lounge
4. gift shop	8. Operating Room	12. fire extinguisher

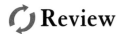 Review

Dialogue Review

Review the dialogue on pages 147–48. As you read, follow the directions. Then compare your answers with a partner.

- Underline the **Prepositions**.
- Circle the **Ask for and Give Directions** phrases.
- Box the **Complex Way to Give Directions**.

Role Plays: Getting around the Facility

Work with a partner. Read each situation, and develop a dialogue to perform for the class.

1. An elderly man is looking for his wife's room. A nurse at the nurse's station explains that she has been moved to the I.C.U. and gives directions.

2. The cafeteria is closed. A man wants to find some food. He asks an environmental services worker if the hospital has vending machines and where they are.

3. A woman needs to find the hospital cashier. A staff member points to the cashier's window.

4. A man wants to know if there's an A.T.M. available. He asks at the reception desk.

5. A nurse tells a family member to go to a waiting area and explains where it is.

6. A woman is looking for the outpatient pharmacy. A security officer gives directions.

7. An elderly woman asks where the chapel is. A nurse's aide directs her.

End-of-Unit Discussion

Sharing

Discuss the questions with a small group.

1. Which part of a hospital seems to be the most confusing? Why?

2. Is it easy or difficult to give directions in a hospital? Why?

3. Discuss some major differences between two medical centers that you are familiar with.

4. If you could design a hospital, what features would you include in all of the nurse's stations?

Culture Point: Giving Feedback

Read this story. Discuss in small groups and as a class.

Two CNAs did a good job setting up a conference room for a training workshop. Their supervisor came into the room to check their work.

Supervisor: Good job. Now let me tell you about tomorrow's schedule. Tomorrow we need to prepare the maternity ward for. . . .

CNA: Excuse me, Ms. White. How could we do a better job with this area?

Supervisor: Everything's fine. Now about tomorrow. . . .

The CNAs were confused by their supervisor's words. Why?

UNIT 9: Being Safe on the Job

Many things can go wrong at a medical facility. Even though there are safety procedures in place, accidents and emergencies still occur. Understanding the influence of safety is important. After an accident, a quick and clear response is needed. Many times this is a report of the accident over the loudspeaker or telephone.

Managing Accidents

If you see something unsafe about to happen, you need to warn somebody. There are many ways to warn someone not to do something or to alert them. You can use your voice to help the words sound serious.

Listening to the Action

 ### Listening for Language

Listen to the conversations between health care workers and family members. What words do the health care workers use to warn the family members.

1. _____

2. _____

3. _____

⇅ Dialogue

Practicing the Language

A nursing assistant is walking by a room when a client has an accident. Practice the dialogue with a partner.

Client: Oh, my! Ouch! Ohh!

Nursing Assistant: Oh, no! Are you O.K.?

Client: Well, I'm alive, but not alive and well.

Nursing Assistant: What happened?

Client: I was enjoying the peace and quiet, and then I decided to go to the bathroom. As I walked across the room, I slipped and fell.

Nursing Assistant: You need to watch out, and go slowly but surely.

Client: Nice and easy, right?

Nursing Assistant: That's right. Here, let me help you to the bathroom.

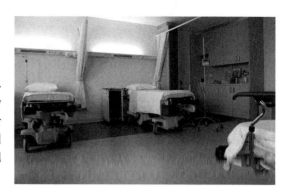 Vocabulary

Word Partnerships

Some words in English commonly appear together. Native speakers use these often and can easily understand the meaning of a phrase when they hear them. Some of these may relate to situations found in a medical facility. Read this list of common word partnerships

alive and well	slip and fall
back and forth	slowly but surely
day in and day out	sooner or later
leaps and bounds	spick and span
nice and easy	step by step
once and for all	ups and downs
out and about	wait and see
peace and quiet	word for word

Matching Word Partnerships

Match the word partnership in the left column with the definition in the right column.

1. _____ alive and well

2. _____ once and for all

3. _____ out and about

4. _____ slowly but surely

5. _____ sooner or later

6. _____ spick and span

a. something will happen only once more and then will stay the same into the future

b. take your time and do a careful job

c. a person is still living and doing fine

d. going to various places and doing things

e. very clean

f. will definitely happen in the future, but the exact time is not certain

Dialogue Completion

Complete the conversations with a word partnerships from the list on page 154.

1. *Client:*   I think my condition is improving quite rapidly, don't you think?

   Nurse: Absolutely! You're improving by _____.

2. *Nurse:*   I've been walking _____ in this ward all day. I could really use a rest.

   Nursing Assistant: I hear ya!

3. *Client:*   Can you turn that machine off? I need some _____.

   Nurse: We'll be finished with this procedure in a moment.

4. *Visitor:*   I really like how the rooms in this hospital are _____.

   Nurse: Yes, well, hospitals need to be germ-free, right?

⇆ Communication Strategy

Giving Warnings

Being safe means keeping your eyes open for yourself and other people. If there is something dangerous going on, you must give a warning. Anything can happen if we are not safe. Some things happen even if we are safe. If something happens, you need to act quickly. You do not want anyone to get injured.

Examples of dangers include falls, spills, slips, trips, incorrect lifts, or needle sticks.

All areas of a medical facility could have hazards. If things are not properly in place, it could be dangerous. Hazards could injure you, other health care workers, or even clients. If you see a hazard, you need to give a warning. Examples of hazards include loose cords, syringes left in a wastebasket, something on the floor, things stacked too high, something blocking the hallway, or open chemical containers.

To be safe in all situations, you need to learn the correct warnings in English.

Dangerous Happenings
   Danger!
   Look out!
   Move out of the way!
   Watch out!

Hazards
   Be careful!
   Be safe.
   Go slowly, please.
   Nice and easy.
   That's dangerous!
   Work safely.

Giving Warnings

Read each situation, and choose the best warning from the box on page 155 or write one of your own.

What do you say to a person who is . . .

1. not lifting something properly? _____

2. about to trip on a cord across the floor? _____   _____

3. trying to pull a book from the middle of a tall stack? _____

4. whose hand is near a wastebasket full of syringes? _____

5. about to walk into a stretcher in a hallway? _____

6. standing near a container of biohazardous chemicals? _____

7. walking near a puddle on the floor? _____

⇄ Communication Strategy

Reporting an Accident or Event

These phrases deal with reporting an accident and then requesting action. Reporting should happen before requesting action or assistance.

Reporting an accident or event

Accident in room _____.

Accident in _____ (space/area).

Accident on _____.

Explosion/fire in _____.

Accident with _____.

Reporting injured persons

No persons injured.

Number of injured persons: _____.

Requesting action

Provide first aid immediately.

Take immediate action to _____.

Requesting assistance

Medical assistance required.

No assistance required.

Technical assistance required.

_____ persons required.

_____ assistance required.

Sentence Completion

Complete the reports with an appropriate word or phrase from the box on page 156.

1. There was an _____ in Room 212.

2. One _____ was injured.

3. First _____ was provided.

4. No additional _____ required.

Writing Reports

Talk about what types of situations might require these reports. Then decide on an appropriate response for each.

Accident Report: _____

Injured Persons Report: _____

Event Report: _____

 # Pronunciation: Rhythm

Rhythm means that there are patterns of stressed words in English sentences. Look at this nursery rhyme. The stressed words are marked. Each line has four equal beats and that pattern creates a "song."

　　•　　•　　•　　　　•
Row, row, row your boat

　•　　　　•　　　•
Gently down the stream.

　•　　　　•　　　•　　　•
Merrily, merrily, merrily, merrily,

•　　　•　　　•
Life is just a dream.

Normal conversations also have rhythm. If you listen carefully, you can hear the "songs" in everyday speech.

　　　　　•　　•　　•
Client: Will I get better soon?

　　　　　•　　•　　　•
Nurse: You'll have your ups and downs.

　　　•　　•　　　•
Client: I want only leaps and bounds.

　　　•　　•　　•
Nurse: We'll have to wait and see.

Rule: Rhythm is possible in English because many words are not stressed. The number of stressed words (and the rhythm) stays the same even when sentences get longer.

Each of these sentences has three stressed words and three beats (• • •).

• • •
Nurses help clients.

• • •
Nurses help the clients.

' ı ▪
The nurses help the clients.

• • •
The nurses will help the clients.

• • •
The nurses will have helped the clients.

• • •
People have accidents.

• • •
People have some accidents.

• • ▪
The people have some accidents.

• • •
The people can have some accidents.

• • •
The people can have some small accidents.

Rhythm

Mark the words that should be stressed.

1. *Home Health Aide:* Don't get up.

   Client: Why not?

   Home Health Aide: The floor is still wet.

   Client: Then, bedpan, please.

   Home Health Aide: Sure thing.

2. *Head Nurse:*   Incoming accident victim!

   Cuts and a broken leg.

   Let's transfer him to the bed.

   On 1, 2, 3.

   Nurse: How did you get so banged up?

   Client: My new skateboard!

3. *Nurse 1:*   We've been so busy all day and all night.

   Accidents and emergencies have kept us awake.

   Nurse 2:   When your shift is over, what will you do?

   Nurse 1:   Go home, take a bath, and read a good book.

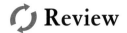 # Review

Dialogue Review

Review the dialogue on page 153. As you read, follow the directions. Then compare your answers with a partner.

- Underline the **Word Partnerships**.
- Circle the **Warnings**.

Role Plays: Accidents

Work with a partner. Read each situation, and develop a dialogue to perform for the class.

1. A client falls out of the bed. A nurse helps and then reports the accident via the phone to the chief nursing officer.

2. An I.V. bag splits and spills chemicals onto the client. A nursing student runs down the hall to find someone and then reports the accident.

3. A supervisor notices a hazard in the hallway and warns a nurse.

4. A client worries about her progress. A home health aide encourages her.

5. A young client slams her finger in the drawer. A nursing assistant reports the accident to a supervisor.

6. One nurse sees a puddle on the floor in the middle of the nurses' work station. Another nurse is about to walk through it. The first nurse warns her.

7. A nurse sees a pediatric client playing with electrical cords next to his bed. She warns the client this is dangerous.

Handling Emergencies

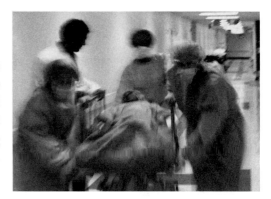

Emergencies can happen anywhere, and they are always serious. Even though there are many plans to handle emergencies when they occur, it is always good to know how and be prepared to react. You should also know how to communicate appropriately during a stressful event like an emergency. Health care workers use special codes for emergency situations.

Listening to the Action

 Listening for Language

Listen to the conversations between health care workers. What codes do they call?

1. _____

2. _____

3. _____

⇅ Dialogue

Practicing the Language

A nurse is reporting an emergency to a supervising nurse. Practice the dialogue with a partner.

Nurse: We have a Code Gray in Room 601!

Supervising Nurse: Did you say Code Gray?

Nurse: Yes, Code Gray!

Supervising Nurse: Is the client under control?

Nurse: Yes, the client is under control. The visitor is out of control.

Supervising Nurse: Instruction: Maintain visual contact. We will get security there A.S.A.P.

Nurse: O.K., I will maintain visual contact.

Supervising Nurse: Is the visitor violent?

Nurse: Yes, the visitor is violent. He is breaking things in the room.

Supervising Nurse: Help is on the way. Stay calm.

Nurse: I'll do my best.

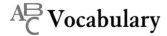 Vocabulary

Emergency Codes

Even though there are efforts being made to standardize code colors, codes can vary by location. Health care workers need to learn the codes at their facilities. Some sample emergency codes are listed.

- Colors:

    Code Amber: child abduction

    Code Blue: a patient needs immediate resuscitation

    Code Gray: an unruly patient or visitor

    Code Green: evacuation

    Code Pink: biohazardous contamination

    Code Purple: psychiatric emergency

    Code Red: incoming life-threatening trauma; fire

    Code Silver: violent situation

    Code Yellow: a bomb threat

- Others:

    Code Rainbow: large-scale disaster or riot

    Code Elope: a client who leaves unannounced

    Code Zebra: bioterrorism

    Dr. Allcome: serious emergency, everybody who is not busy must "come"

    Dr. Firestone: fire in the hospital

Sentence Completion

Complete the sentences with the correct emergency code. Some sentences may have more than one answer.

1. If we have a _____, we need to call the bomb squad.

2. Nancy had to call a _____ during the last shift because a man came in with a knife.

3. When our ward had a _____, a nurse used a fire extinguisher to put it out.

4. It is not easy for clients to leave, but sometimes a _____ must be called.

5. I heard that we had a _____ last year when that baby was taken from the maternity ward.

Code Identifying

What code would you call for each situation?

1. A client's heart has stopped. = Code _____

2. A client with mental problems needs help. = Code _____

3. Fourteen rival gang members are fighting in the ED. = Code ___ ___

4. A tornado has caused many seriously injured clients to arrive. = Code _____

5. Everyone needs to leave the facility. = Code _____

⇆ Communication Strategy

Responding

There may be times when you have to call someone for assistance during an emergency. The emergency personnel could give you important advice or instructions to do something quickly. This communication should always be simple and clear. It is a good idea to repeat the important phrases when you are responding to instructions.

When the answer to a question is affirmative

Yes, _____.

A: "Is the third floor secure?"
B: "Yes, the third floor is secure."

When the answer to a question is negative

No, _____.

A: "Is client under control?"
B: "No, the client is not under control."

When the information requested is not immediately available

"Stand by."

A: "Are there injured persons?"
B: "Stand by. We will know in five minutes."

When the information requested cannot be obtained

"No information."

A: "Is the pathway clear?"
B: "No information."

Dialogue Practice

Read and practice the dialogues with a partner.

1. *Nurse:*   Fire in the cafeteria!

   Security Officer: What's on fire?

   Nurse: The grill and surrounding area.

   Security Officer: Secure the area.

   Nurse: Yes, I'll secure the area now.

2. *Nurse:*   Chemical spill near the activities room!

   Emergency Worker: Location?

   Nurse: Between the south end exit and the elevator.

   Emergency Worker: Report injured persons.

   Nurse: No persons injured.

   Emergency Worker: Seal off area immediately.

   Nurse: Yes, I will seal off area immediately.

3. *Nurse:*   Reporting a possible broken neck.

   Doctor: Is the victim lying down?

   Nurse: Yes, the victim is lying down.

   Doctor: Keep the head stabilized.

   Nurse: Yes, I'll keep the head stabilized.

Dialogue Completion

Complete the dialogues with an appropriate response to the questions.

1. Is the client stable? _____

2. Is the ED secure? _____

3. Is the activity room all clear of clients? _____

⇆ Communication Strategy

Following Phone Conversations

It can be difficult to understand a caller because you can't see facial expressions or gestures. You might have to ask the caller to repeat or clarify information.

If you're not sure that you understand

Did you say . . . ?
Are you saying . . . ?
(Do) you mean . . . ?

If you believe that you understand

O.K., you said that
So what you're saying is,
O.K., I got it.

General requests to clarify

I didn't get that.
I'm sorry. I didn't understand.
Would you mind saying that again?
Could you please repeat that?

Specific requests to clarify

Excuse me. To whom do you wish to speak?
Pardon? I didn't get your name.
Could you repeat just the last part?

Dialogue Completion

Complete the following telephone conversations with appropriate phrases from the box on page 164. Then read and practice them with a partner.

1. *Nurse:* The storm damage has blocked any pathway out of the 4th floor!

   Responder: Stay put. Emergency crews are on the way.

   Nurse: _____ that I should stand by before help arrives?

   Responder: Yes. There is nothing we can do before this.

   Nurse: O.K. We will manage.

2. *Nurse:* Cardiac Recovery. May I help you?

   Caller: Yes, I'm calling to check on the results from an ultrasound.

   Nurse: _____? _____. You need results for what?

   Caller: Ultrasound.

   Nurse: I'm sorry, you've called the wrong number. I will transfer you to the Ultrasound Lab now.

3. *Nurse:* This is Outpatient Oncology. How may I be of service?

   Caller: Hi. I need to speak to Dr. Thurber.

   Nurse: Excuse me._____?

   Caller: Dr. Thurber, please.

   Nurse: Yes, Dr. Thurber. He is out to lunch now. He will return at 2:00 PM.

   Caller: Thank you. I will call back then.

Pronunciation: Reduced Speech (Verbs)

In English, reduced speech (fast speech) is most often used in informal conversations, but it can also be used in formal situations. Sometimes reduced speech is used with verbs. In an emergency, fast speech is common because everyone is working quickly. Listen to your instructor read the examples.

Slow speech		Reduced speech
I'm going to go.	→	I'm **gonna** go.
I want to go.	→	I **wanna** go
I have to go.	→	I **hafta** go.
She has to go.	→	She **hasta** go.
I've got to go.	→	I've **gotta** go.
I could have gone.	→	I **coulda** gone.
I would have gone.	→	I **woulda** gone.
I should have gone.	→	I **shoulda** gone.

Recognizing Reduced Speech

Complete the dialogues with an appropriate reduced word. Then practice with a partner.

1. *ED Nurse:*   Incoming train accident victim. Nearly severed foot. She _____ be taken to bay 1.

   ED Doctor: I'm _____ need a foot specialist. Call Dr. Prabhu.

2. *New Nurse:*   The victims keep coming and coming. I _____ help them all, but there's so many!

   Nurse: You just _____ concentrate on one at a time. One at a time.

3. *Security Guard:* You've _____ calm down, Sir!

   Client: I think I'm _____ die.

   Security Guard: O.K., we'll find a doctor right away!

Practicing Reduced Speech

Think of things in your life that you could have done, would have done, or should have done. Complete the sentences, and then share your answers with the class. Use reduced speech. The first one has been done for you as an example.

1. This morning *I coulda temporarily worked in the vascular center.* _____

2. This morning _____.

3. Last year _____.

4. Last week _____.

5. If I had known, _____.

6. If I had known, _____.

7. When I was young, _____.

8. When I was young, _____.

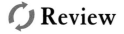 # Review

Dialogue Review

Review the dialogue on page 160. As you read, follow the directions. Then compare your answers with a partner.

- Underline the **Emergency Code** terms.
- Circle the **Responding** phrases.
- Box the **Follow a Conversation** phrase.

Role Plays: Emergencies

Work with a partner. Read each situation, and develop a dialogue to perform for the class.

1. A nurse in the ED answers the phone. The caller is angry at a doctor. He says, "The doctor let my daughter die." The caller says that there is a bomb somewhere in the hospital.

2. A psychiatric client starts to hallucinate and scream. Two nurses see this happen and decide to call a Code Purple.

3. A person who speaks only a little English calls a large medical center and asks to speak to one person. The staff member must use many requests for repetitions and clarifications.

4. A 60-year-old man is choking in the parking lot. An environmental services worker calls a doctor to respond to the emergency.

5. A 5.5 earthquake occurs. Visitors and staff members start running out of the hospital. A nurse from the fifth floor calls the main desk to report the status on her floor.

6. Two nurses see syringes in a small wastebasket and discuss if they can empty it or if they should call the sanitation team.

7. Someone calls 9-1-1 to report that the city is being attacked by martians. The 9-1-1 operator checks to make sure he understood correctly.

End-of-Unit Discussion

Sharing

Discuss the questions with a small group.

1. Which type of accidents do you think cause the most injuries?

2. Have you ever had to report an accident? What information did you give?

3. Do you think that all emergency codes should be standard in all English-speaking countries? What are the dangers of having different codes at different hospitals?

4. Do you like communicating over the phone? Which type of information is the hardest to catch over the telephone?

Culture Point: Giving Praise

Read this story. Discuss in small groups and then as a class.

—————

Nurse Melanie had been working in the United States for a few months as a pediatric nurse. One day, Melanie discovered that a teenager who was visiting his baby brother started a fire in a trash container. She ran to get a fire extinguisher and put it out. She was chosen as the Employee of the Month for her workplace. Her supervisor happily told her that she would receive an award from the president of the hospital at a ceremony.

—————

Melanie is upset by this news. Why?

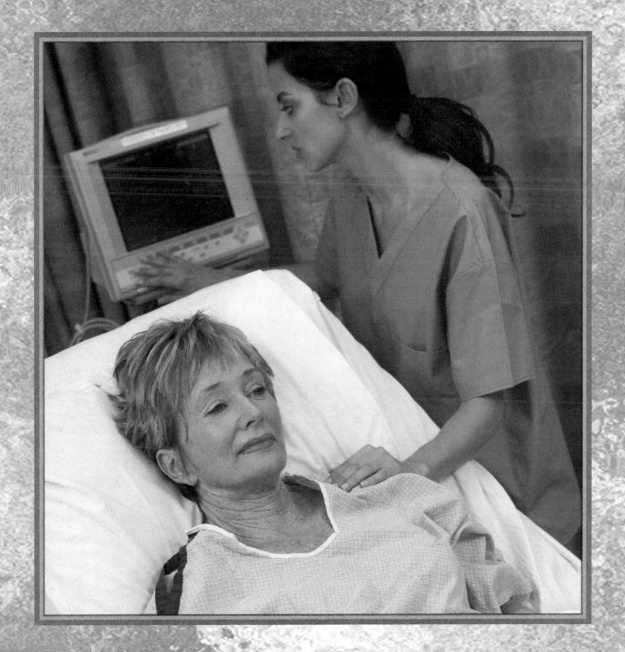

PART 5

Caring for Clients

UNIT 10: Providing Assistance

Health care workers provide many services for their clients. Many times they have to help with something physical. They might have to move clients, help clean, or give instructions. It is necessary to kindly offer this help with verbal intentions followed by clear instructions and check for understanding. If all these communication skills are used, the client will experience smooth and comfortable care.

Giving Instructions

It is very important to make instructions as simple as possible so they can be understood. Some clients may be in pain, distracted, or may not hear well. There are some basic principles for effective communication with clients. Health care workers need to remember these when helping the client do something or when conducting any procedure.

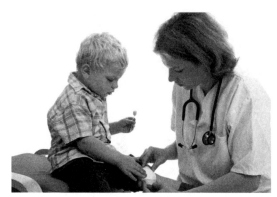

- explain the procedure
- check for understanding
- seek cooperation
- encourage the client
- reassure the client
- give feedback

Listening to the Action

 Listening for Language

Listen to the conversations between health care workers and clients. What phrases do the health care workers use to explain steps in procedure in Conversation 1, check for understanding in Conversation 2, and reassure in Conversation 3?

1. _____

2. _____

3. _____

⇅ Dialogue

Practicing the Language

A client with a hip injury needs to be turned in bed. A nurse is giving instructions. Practice the dialogue with a partner.

Nurse: Hello, Mr. Folse. How is your hip doing? That was quite an injury you sustained: a broken hip and a dislocated knee.

Client: Yes. I am lucky to be alive. I still feel some swelling here.

Nurse: Well, it's time to roll you over. We don't want you to get bed sores from lying in one position.

Client: Is it going to hurt? Last time I felt a sharp pain.

Nurse: Don't worry. We will take it easy and do it together, step by step. First, I'll have you cross your arms across your chest. Good. Next, I'll gently move your upper body toward me. Then, I'll do the middle part and lower part. Are you following me?

Client: Yes, I am. Are you then going to flip me?

Nurse: Not yet. I need to get some assistance for that.

Client: Oh, boy. I'm really nervous.

Nurse: Everything will be fine. Here comes Juanita. We will be very gentle. Here we go, Mr. Folse. Please take a deep breath and relax.

ᴬᴮ𝒞 Vocabulary

Common Injuries and Related Words

Even though there are hundreds of different injuries, knowing the most common ones will be useful in your career.

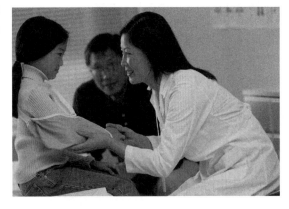

- **Common Injuries:** bed sore, bruise, broken (bone), bump, burn, cut/laceration, dislocated elbow, gash, graze, lesion, sprain, tear, wound/puncture wound

- **Related Words:** boil, cyst, growth, lump, infection, rash, scab, spot, swollen (leg), inflamed (ankle)

Sentence Completion

Complete the sentences with an injury or related word from page 171.

1. A _____ is an injury that results in a break or opening in the skin.

2. A _____ shoulder is when a bone is pushed or pulled out of position.

3. When a ligament is stretched too far or tears, the joint will become painful and swollen. The diagnosis is a

4. A _____ is blood collected underneath the skin and is caused by trauma to an area of the body.

5. A _____ is the result of inflammation and damage caused by irritation to the skin and slowed blood flow. It happens when someone is in the same position in bed for a long time.

Categorizing

Name three body parts for each category.

1. Body parts that can break

   _____   _____   _____

2. Body parts that can swell

   _____   _____   _____

3. Body parts that can be fractured

   _____   _____   _____

4. Body parts that can dislocated

   _____   _____   _____

⇆ Communication Strategy

Checking for Understanding

When you need to know that someone understands you, use extra phrases. There are many phrases to use to determine if a client, another health care worker, or a doctor can understand you. You must be careful to use the appropriate form (formal or informal) when checking comprehension.

Formal

> Pardon me. Can you understand what I said?
>
> Excuse me. Am I making myself clear?
>
> I'm sorry. Am I making sense?
>
> Sorry. Are you following me?

Informal

> Am I making sense?
>
> Are you following me?
>
> Can you understand me?
>
> Is that clear?

Dialogue Practice

Read and practice the dialogue with a partner.

1. *Nurse:*   I need you to roll over to the side, please.

   Client: Hmm.

   Nurse: Sorry. Are you following me?

   Client: Oh, yeah. Something . . . the side?

   Nurse: Right. I need you to roll over to the side.

2. *Supervising Nurse:* You need to give Mr. Vortis his antibiotic through the I.V.

   Nurse: Give antibiotics, right?

   Supervising Nurse: Am I making myself clear?

   Nurse: Oh, sure. Antibiotics through his I.V.

Dialogue Completion

Complete the dialogues with phrases from the box on page 173. Then read and practice the dialogues with a partner.

1. *Nurse:*   When should I attend to the transfusion client in 210-B?

   Head Nurse: Yes.

   Nurse: _____. _____?

   Head Nurse: Oh. Can you repeat that, then?

   Nurse: When should I attend to the transfusion client in Room 210-B?

   Head Nurse: Oh, right away, please.

   Nurse: O.K. No problem.

2. *Nurse 1:*   Can I get an update on Ms. Belcher's blood pressure?

   Nurse 2:   Huh?

   Nurse 1:   _____?

   Nurse 2:   I think so. Ms. Belcher in 1209-A, right?

   Nurse 1:   Yes, that's right.

   Nurse 2:   Right away.

3. *Nurse:*   Please sit up for your sponge bath, O.K.?

   Sleepy Client: Sponge bad?

   Nurse: _____?

   Sleepy Client: No, not really.

   Nurse: We need you to sit up for your sponge bath now. Is that O.K. with you?

   Sleepy Client: Sure. That sounds good.

⇆ Communication Strategy

Giving Instructions

Many times instructions are given step by step. They have a clear beginning, middle, and end and each step must be done in sequence. When you are giving good instructions, you need to make each step clear. Use a word from each column to tell what happens step by step.

Beginning	Middle	End
First	Second	Finally
At the beginning	After	At last
At first	Next	The final step
Step 1	Then	The last step
	The next step	
	Step 2, 3, 4	

Dialogue Practice

Read and practice the dialogue with a partner.

Nurse: Hello, Mr. Wilson. We need to change the dressing on your wound.

Client: Can you tell me what you will do?

Nurse: Sure. First, I'll place the supplies on a sterile metal tray. Second, I'll open the packages and lay the bandages out. Then, I'll wash my hands and put on a pair of latex gloves. Next, I'll gently peel back and remove the old dressing and throw it away using tweezers. Then, I'll check your wound to see if it is healing well. Next, I'll apply a sterile nonstick gauze pad and more dressing with tape. Finally, I'll throw away used material and wash my hands again.

Client: Thanks for explaining it to me.

Explaining a Procedure

Choose two situations, and write step-by-step directions with a partner. Add more lines if necessary.

| answer a call light | change shifts | strip discharge beds |
| assess a patient | collect a urine sample | transfer a resident |

How to: _____

A: Excuse me. I want to _____

What do I have to do?

B: Well, first, _____

A: OK. Then what?

B: Then, _____

A: I see. What's next?

B: Next, _____

A: I _____? Is that all?

B: Well, finally you have to _____

Pronunciation: Contrastive Stress

Contrastive stress is stressing one word more than another. Listen to your instructor read the examples. Which words get more stress? Why?

> •   •   •   •   •
>
> *Nurse 1:* His parents were excited to see him get up out of bed.

> •   •   •   • • •
>
> *Nurse 2:* Yes, but they were really excited to see him walk 50 steps!

> •   •   •   •   •
>
> *Nurse 1:* It's Sunday, so maybe the ED won't be busy this evening.

> • •   •   •   •   •   •
>
> *Nurse 2:* It's Super Bowl Sunday, so the ED will definitely be busy this evening!

In the first example, both speakers use the word *excited,* but Nurse 2 says *really excited. Really* is new information, so it gets more stress. Nurse 1 says, "Get up out of bed," and then Nurse 2 says, "Walk 50 steps." *walk 50 steps* is different information, so it gets more stress.

In the second example, Nurse 2 is correcting Nurse 1. It is not a regular Sunday; it's Super Bowl Sunday, and the prediction is that it will be busy.

<u>Rule</u>: Use contrastive stress when the word gives new information, different information, or corrected information.

Recognizing Contrastive Stress

Read the dialogues. Mark the word or words in the responses that should be stressed more than the others.

1. *Nurse 1:* I've worked for Mission Hospital for three years.

   Nurse 2: Really? I've worked for Mission Hospital for five years.

2. *Nurse 1:* The floor is really quiet today.

   Nurse 2: I bet the whole ward is really quiet too.

3. *Nurse 1:* Are you upset?

   Nurse 2: No, I'm tired.

4. *Nurse 1:* Tomorrow my shift starts at 7:00 AM.

   Nurse 2: No, tomorrow your shift starts at 6:00 AM.

Making Corrections

Read the sentences, and then correct the mistakes. Mark the words that should receive more stress. Practice them with a partner. The first one has been done for you as an example.

1. Young patients are in the geriatrics center.

   •

   No, they're in the pediatrics center.

2. The president of the medical staff is the highest position in this hospital.

3. First degree burns are worse than second degree burns.

4. Do I fold the washcloth first and then wipe?

5. A bruise can often turn pink.

Adding New Information

Answer the questions, and add new requests. Practice them with a partner. The first one has been done for you as an example.

1. Do you need some bandages? Yes, but I need clips too.

2. Would you like me to get more towels? _____.

3. Can I get you some cotton balls? _____.

4. Will you need some antiseptic? _____.

5. Would you like more light? _____.

6. Are you going to need more gauze? _____.

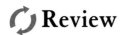 # Review

Dialogue Review

Review the dialogue on page 171. As you read, follow the directions. Then compare your answers with a partner.

- Underline the **Injury** terms.
- Circle the **Giving Instruction** phrases.
- Box the **Checking for Understanding** phrase.

Role Plays: Giving Instructions

Work with a partner. Read each situation, and develop a dialogue to perform for the class.

A nurse is teaching the following procedures to a client. The client is giving verbal cues. The nurse can check for understanding.

1. emptying and changing a urinary drainage bag

2. bathing (partial or complete bed bath, tub bath, shower, or perineal care)

3. dressing or undressing

4. using a self-operated pain drip

5. changing a dressing on a wound

6. getting out of bed

7. ambulating (cane, walker, or gait belt)

Providing Everyday Needs

Different clients need different care. Many of them, though, need to be bathed or fed. Health care workers offer to help in a variety of ways. It can be challenging to provide this assistance. Health care workers need to be clear about what they intend to do. It can make clients more comfortable if they know what will happen next.

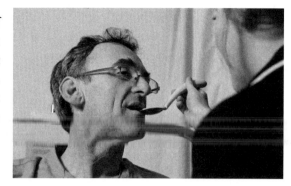

Listening to the Action

Listening for Language

Listen to the conversations between health care workers and clients. What phrases do the health care workers use to show intention to offer help?

1. _____

2. _____

3. _____

⇅ Dialogue

Practicing the Language

A client has just woken up and realized she had a BM. A nurse offers help. Practice the dialogue with a partner.

Nurse: Good morning, Mrs. Carr! How are we today?

Client: Oh, fine, I guess.

Nurse: I intend to change your disposable briefs and then clean you up a bit. I'll wash your hair and clip your nails. Is that O.K. with you?

Client: Yes. Thank you. I think I did some business last night.

Nurse: Fine. Do you need some assistance sitting up?

Client: No, thanks. I can manage.

Nurse: All right, now, may I please help you take off your robe?

Client: Yes.

Nurse: I'm going to bathe you now. Did you sleep well last night?

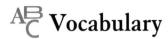 # Vocabulary

Personal Hygiene

Excellent personal hygiene must be practiced at all times. Health care workers should take care of clothes, hair, hands, and nails. They should not use strong scented products. Hands must be washed thoroughly several times a day. The list contains common personal hygiene terms.

- **Nouns**

    Body: anti-perspirant, body soap, cologne/perfume, deodorant, facial soap, liquid soap

    Face: aftershave lotion, electric shaver, razor blade, moisturizer

    Hair: brush, comb, conditioner/rinse, curling iron, hair dryer, hair gel, hairspray, shampoo

    Hands: lotion, nail clippers, nail file/emery board

    Mouth: cleanser, dental floss, mouthwash, toothpaste, toothbrush

    Perineal: disposable briefs, feminine hygiene products (tampon/sanitary napkin/douche)

- **Verbs:** bathe, brush (one's hair), brush (one's teeth), clip/file (one's nails), comb, dry, floss, shampoo

Multiple Choice

Circle the best answer for each sentence.

1. Can we help you use your **dental floss / mouthwash** today?

2. I took a shower and forgot to use **perfume / shampoo** on my hair.

3. I see that someone didn't use **facial soap / liquid soap.** Look at her fingers.

4. Mr. Kay's dentures need to be soaked in **cleanser / aftershave.**

5. This facility does not have a **nail file / curling iron** to do your hair like that.

Sentence Completion

Complete each sentence with a word or phrase from the list at the top of the page.

1. Your hair looks so nice. Did you use _____?

2. The client prefers to trim her own nails. Can you get the _____?

3. Nurse, I need some _____. My husband will be coming to visit soon, and I'm afraid that I don't smell very good right now.

4. You'll have to use an _____, Mr. Herrera. This facility doesn't allow clients to use razor blades.

5. That client's skin is dry. Please bring a supply of _____ to her bathroom.

⇆ Communication Strategy

Offering Help

There will be many times when a client needs your help. Good communication starts with a verbal offer to help this person. Of course, part of everyone's job is to offer help to clients, so using the appropriate phrases will allow the clients to understand you better.

Formal

> (How) may I help you?
> May I be of service to you?
> Would you like me to help you?

Less Formal

> Can I help you?
> Do you need some help?
> How about letting me help you?
> Let me give you a hand
> Let me help you.

If someone offers to help you, you can either accept or refuse their help. Rejections should be polite by including some sort of expression of gratitude. If possible, a rejection should include an explanation.

Ways to Accept Help

> That's nice of you, thanks.
> That would be great. Thanks.
> If you don't mind.
> Please.

Ways to Reject Help

> No, but I appreciate the offer.
> No, it's all right. I can (do it myself/manage).
> Thanks (a lot), but I'm fine.
> No, but thanks anyway.

Dialogue Practice

Read and practice the dialogues with a partner.

1. *Nurse:*   Excuse me, Miss. How about letting me help you put on your socks?
   Client: That would be great. Thanks. I really can't bend over well.

2. *Nurse 1:*   Do you need some help with Mr. Corolla?
   Nurse 2:   No, it's all right. I can manage.

3. *Nurse:*   Would you like me to help you, sir?
   Client: Thanks a lot, but I'm fine.

4. *Nurse:*   Can I help you cut your meat?
   Client: If you don't mind.

Writing Offers of Help

Write an offer of help for each situation.

1. You see a client trying to reach something that is too high to reach easily.

   _____.

2. A client needs to ambulate.

   _____.

3. A client has severe back pain and might need a back rub.

   _____.

4. Another nurse is trying to give a bed bath to a restless client.

   _____.

⇆ Communication Strategy

Stating Intentions

When you plan to do something for clients, it is a good idea to tell them in advance. This is called **stating your intention.** This will lower stress because the person you are working with knows what will happen next. He or she will be prepared, and the process should go more smoothly. There are several ways to state your intentions.

I am determined to (get you feeling better).

I intend to (bathe you before your family comes).

I'm going to (help you get out of bed).

I'm planning to (feed you some gelatin).

I've decided to (lower your level of pain medication).

Clients can state intentions as well.

I am determined to (get better quickly).

I intend to (go through a successful operation).

I'm going to (quit smoking).

I'm planning to (go on vacation when I get out of here).

I've decided to (change my eating habits).

Dialogue Practice

Read and practice the dialogues with a partner.

1. *Nurse:*   Mr. Landers, I'm going to show you how to re-wrap your knee.

   Client: Will I have to do this every day?

   Nurse: No. You need to do this procedure every other day.

2. *Visitor:*   Now that you are feeling better, what do you plan on changing in your life?

   Client: I am determined to watch my sugar intake.

   Visitor: Good. The doctor says that your diabetes will only get worse if you don't.

3. *Nurse:*   I intend to change your pants now, Mr. Rogers. Is that fine with you?

   Client: Well, if you insist.

   Nurse: I insist. O.K., after this I am planning to shave you. Do you prefer an electric razor?

Writing Intentions

Complete the following intentions with a procedure for a client or a plan of your own. Then share your answers with a small group.

1. I am determined to _____

2. I've decided to _____

3. I'm going to _____

4. I intend to _____

5. I'm planning to _____

Pronunciation: *can* vs. *can't*

The pronunciation of the vowel sound in *can* and *can't* varies. Listen to your instructor read the short answers. Does the vowel sound the same?

> Yes, I can.
> No, I can't.

<u>Rule</u>: When we say *can* and *can't* in short answers, the pronunciation of the vowel *a* is the same. We use the /æ/ sound. It's long and clear, and we stress the word.

Listen to your instructor read these statements. How does the pronunciation change?

- Affirmative statement: *I can walk to the bathroom by myself.*
- Affirmative question: *Can you walk to the bathroom by yourself?*
- Affirmative long answer: *Yes, I can walk to the bathroom by myself.*

<u>Rule</u>: In saying *can* in affirmative statements, affirmative questions, and long answers, the pronunciation of the vowel *a* is different. We use a schwa sound /ə/. It is very short, and we do not stress the word.

Listen to your instructor read these examples.

- Negative statement: *I can't walk to the bathroom by myself.*
- Negative question: *Can't you walk to the bathroom by yourself?*
- Negative long answer: *No, I can't walk to the bathroom by myself.*

<u>Rule</u>: For the *can't* in negative statements, negative questions and long answers, use the /æ/ sound. It's long and clear, and we stress the word.

Practicing *can* and *can't*

Make a list of nursing procedures that you can and cannot do right now in your career as a health care worker. Share your answers.

1. I can . . .   *check a client's vital signs.*

   _____ .

   _____ '

   _____ .

2. I can't . . .   *hang I.V. bags.*   _____ .

   _____ .

   _____ .

   _____ .

Using *can* and *can't*

Answer the questions with appropriate information about what the clients can and can't do with personal hygiene. The first one has been done for you as an example.

1. Clients who have ROM difficulties with their arms

   can clip their nails, but can't shampoo their hair. _____

2. Clients who have ROM difficulties with their legs

   _____ .

3. Clients who are allergic to hygiene products with strong scents

   _____ .

4. Clients who must stay in the hospital bed

   _____ .

5. Clients who must not eat or drink anything for eight hours

   _____ .

6. Clients who are about to have surgery

   _____ .

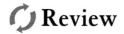 Review

Dialogue Review

Review the dialogue on page 179. As you read, follow the directions. Then compare your answers with a partner.

- Underline the **Personal Hygiene** terms.
- Circle the **Offering Help** phrases.
- Box the **Stating Intentions** phrases.

Role Plays: Everyday Needs

Work with a partner. Read each situation, and develop a dialogue to perform for the class.

1. A client is reaching for a hairbrush on the table next to the bed. A nurse offers help.

2. A young boy looks lost. A nurse offers help and gives directions.

3. An elderly client says that she needs to use the restroom. A nursing assistant offers help.

4. A client is ambulating with you, but she forgot her glasses in her room. A nurse offers help.

5. A restless client is very uncomfortable with the wrist straps. A nurse states the intention to release the client when she calms down.

6. A client isn't eating and looks depressed. The nurse states his intention to help him be well again.

7. A client is very lonely and would like to call her family. The nurse states the intention to help her make a call after the procedure.

End-of-Unit Discussion

Discuss the questions with a small group.

1. Which common injuries have you or your family members had in the past? Did everything heal well?

2. Discuss a very basic procedure that consists of about four or five steps. Does everyone do the steps in the same order or is it possible to vary the order of the steps?

3. In terms of personal hygiene, which things are easiest to do? Which things are hardest to do?

4. Share some of your intentions for the next few months with the group.

Culture Point: Yes and No Answers

Read this story. Discuss in small groups and as a class.

Nurse Victoria was giving Mrs. Aoki instructions on how to give herself insulin injections. Mrs. Aoki appeared to understand the procedure. Victoria then told her that she needed to do it twice a day and checked for comprehension, asking, "Is that clear?" Mrs. Aoki answered, "Yes." The following week, Victoria saw that Mrs. Aoki had only used half of her insulin supply for the week. She realized that she needed to get an interpreter who spoke Mrs. Aoki's native language.

Why was there a miscommunication?

UNIT 11: Monitoring Clients

One of the most important tasks in caring for clients is to monitor them. Clients need to be checked in many ways. Health care workers need to be fluent when speaking about body parts, knowledgeable about symptoms and remedies, and able to keep records on the status of each client throughout the day.

Identifying Symptoms and Remedies

Many problems can occur with the human body. Luckily there are symptoms, or warning signs, that appear to direct health care workers to the best remedy. There may be times when you give minor advice to a client or discuss the options about their treatments. It is important to recognize their symptoms.

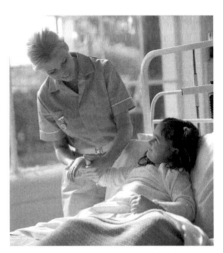

Listening to the Action

Listening for Language

Listen to the conversations between health care workers and clients. What symptoms do the clients mention?

1. _____

2. _____

3. _____

⇅ Dialogue

Practicing the Language

A nurse is talking to a client about her symptoms. Practice the dialogue with a partner.

Nurse: Hello, Mrs. Lynch. My name is Barbara, and I will be your nurse today.

Client: Hello. Barbara is a beautiful name.

Nurse: Thank you. So, you say you have a sore throat, a headache, and chills?

Client: Yes. And my chest feels a little tight. I can't breathe too well.

Nurse: I see. How long has this been going on?

Client: Well, for about three days now. That's why I came in today.

Nurse: I see. Have you eaten anything out of the ordinary recently? I mean, some kind of food that you normally do not eat?

Client: Well, we did go to an Indian restaurant the other day. Besides that, no.

Nurse: Hmmm. It might be caused by a food allergy. What if we did some allergy testing?

Client: That might be good.

Nurse: If I were you, I would get as much rest as possible while you are here.

ABC Vocabulary

Common Medications

In Unit 6, you learned some common abbreviations. Here is a list of some common medications and abbreviations used in medical facilities. Other medication-related terms are included.

Nurses need to make sure they have checked the six rights:

- **Right** client
- **Right** time and frequency of med
- **Right** dose
- **Right** route of administration
- **Right** drug

Review the abbreviations a.c., B.I.D., p.c., Q.I.D., and T.I.D. on page 101. Other common medication, abbreviations, and words and their definitions are listed.

- **Medication Abbreviations**

  as needed = pm   every four hours = q4h

  at night = hs   ointment = ung

  capsule = cap   once a day = QD

  cream = cr   tablet = tab

  day = d

- **Types of Medications**

  antacid—drug used to decrease acid in stomach

  antibiotic—drug used internally to stop or slow growth of germs

  antiseptic—substance used externally to stop or slow down growth of germs

  depressant—drug that slows down the action of the central nervous system

  glucose—sugar found in blood

  tranquilizer—drug used to control anxiety

- **Other Medication Words**

    absorption—the way a drug enters the body

    adverse effect—side effect

    benefit—valued or desired outcome

    efficacy—effectiveness

    fasting—not eating or drinking for set amount of time

    hypodermal—under the skin

    intramuscular (I.M.) injection—injection of a substance into a muscle

    intravenous (I.V.) injection—injection of a substance into a vein

    monitor—check on, keep track of, watch carefully

    sublingual—under the tongue

    tolerance—decrease in response to fixed dosage

    topical application—medication directly on the skin

    toxicity—any harmful effect of a drug or poison

    transdermal—through the skin

Matching

Match the type of drug in the left column with a condition or problem in the right column.

1. tranquilizer _____   a. over active nervous system

2. antibiotic _____   b. cyst on skin exposed to germs

3. antiseptic _____   c. bad stomachache

4. antacid _____   d. nervousness

5. depressant _____   e. internal infection from germs

Sentence Completion

Complete the sentences with the best word from the list on pages 189–90.

1. The nurse said the medication may cause _____.

2. He explained the cream has a _____ because it goes on the skin.

3. The doctor asked us to _____ Mr. Kane since he started a new medicine.

4. That medication requires _____. You can't eat for 12 hours.

6. I think the medicine will work. It has proven _____.

A^B_C Vocabulary

Body Parts

Many people have minor problems with their body. You need to ask clear questions and pronounce the names of the body parts well. You must know the words to express a client's symptoms and give basic advice. The basic body parts are listed.

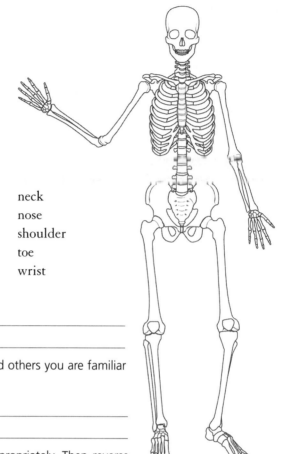

ankle	hand	neck
arm	head	nose
elbow	knee	shoulder
eye	leg	toe
finger	mouth	wrist
foot/feet		

Labeling

Label the skeleton with the names of body parts. Add others you are familiar with.

Dialogue Practice

Using the dialogue as a model, fill in the blanks appropriately. Then reverse roles. Keep practicing with different words.

A: What's the problem?

B: My _____ hurt/hurts.
             (body part)

A: Is it serious?

B: No, I don't think so

A: Do you have any other problems?

B: Yes. I have a(n) _____.
                           (symptom)

A: You should _____.
                              (remedy)

⇆ Communication Strategy

Discussing Options

Sometimes there is a choice of remedies. You may have to discuss the options of doing something one way or the other. It is important to communicate, in an open way, the options. Clients should feel like they have control over some of the decisions when possible. Having an open conversation is a good way to keep a client happy and aware.

Suggesting an option

How about . . . ?

What if we . . .

Would it be possible to . . . ?

Would this be O.K.?

Would this work?

Rejecting an option

I can't imagine doing that.

I don't think that would work.

I'm not sure that is an option.

Accepting an option

That might be good.

That's perfect.

That's possible.

That would work.

Asking to choose an option

Is it better for you (to) _____ or _____?

Would you like (to) _____ or _____?

You have two choices: _____ or _____.

Choosing an option

How about _____?

I want (to) _____.

Well, I think I'd prefer _____.

Nurse: Your knee is swelling. Let's lift it up onto a pillow. Would this be O.K.?

Client: I can't imagine doing that. I'm in too much pain.

Nurse: How about some ice?

Client: That might be good.

Dialogue Practice

Read and practice the dialogues with a partner.

1. *Nurse:*   If your stomach is upset, then what if we gave you an antacid?

   Client: That's perfect.

2. *Nurse:*   We need to change the dressing on your neck area. I have some nice cream to put on it. Would this work for you?

   Client: That would work.

3. *Head Nurse:* We need to give a sedative to Mr. Jones in 213-A.

   Nurse: I'm not sure that is an option. He is allergic to that kind of medication.

   Head Nurse: Oh no. Are you sure? O.K. We need an alternative technique.

Writing Dialogues

Write a short dialogue about the options for each topic with a partner.

1. Take a bath or take a shower.

2. Eat the chicken dinner or the fish dinner.

3. Take more pain medication or do some breathing exercises.

4. Calm down or wear a restraint (for a violent client).

5. Use an oral thermometer or a rectal thermometer.

⇆ Communication Strategy

Giving Advice

You may need to give advice to clients or to other health care workers. Also, a supervisor may sometimes give you advice. Giving advice in English may be strong or weak, depending on the situation. Adding specific words before the verbs, such as *strongly* or *really*, shows that the advice is strong.

I *strongly* suggest that you learn more English.

Although sometimes it is necessary to give direct advice, other times it is not a good idea to give direct advice to a client. This might sound too strong to them. You can soften the message.

Strong/Direct

I suggest/propose/recommend that you

My advice is that you

Less Strong

You should/could/ought to

If I were you, I would

It might be a good idea to

Weak/Softer

You could

Why don't you

You might try to

I sometimes

If someone gives you advice, you can accept it or reject it by using specific phrases. When you reject advice (just like rejecting an invitation), it is polite to not give a reason.

Accepting advice:
All right.
That's a (good / great) idea.
That's a (good / great) suggestion.
Thanks for your advice.
Thanks. I'll do that.

Rejecting advice:
I'm afraid that won't help me because
I can't do that because
I'll think about it.
That's not such a good idea for me because

Dialogue Practice

Read and practice the dialogues with a partner.

1. *Charge Nurse:* Why don't you try doing it this way? I always do that.
   Staff Nurse: That's a good idea. Thanks.

2. *Nurse 1:* I recommend that you request a promotion.
   Nurse 2: That's a good suggestion. I'll do that. Thanks.

3. *Client.* Which food has the most calories? I am trying to gain weight.
   Nurse: I suggest that you order the beef with potatoes.

4. *Nurse:* It might be a good idea to take a walk now.
   Client: I'm afraid I can't do that because I'm in pain.

Giving Advice

Give appropriate advice for each situation.

1. A client is struggling to get dressed.

   _____

2. A nurse is trying to lift too many items onto a cart.

   _____

3. A nurse is trying to lift a client from bed.

   _____

4. A nurse wants to learn to operate a piece of equipment.

   _____

Pronunciation: Linking Consonant to Consonant

In English, words link together to make smooth, connected sentences. If one word ends with a consonant and the next word begins with the same consonant, those two consonants link the words together.

Rule: Two words link together with no silent space between eight consonants.

s	serious swelling	sounds like seriousswelling
l	an abdominal lesion	sounds like an abdominallesion
i	a severe rash	sounds like a severerash
n	a swollen neck	sounds like a swollenneck
m	some moles	sounds like somemoles
f	a stiff finger	sounds like a stiffinger
w	a few welts	sounds like a fewwelts
y	dry eyes	sounds like dryeyes

Rule: With other consonants, the first of the pair is silent, and the second is pronounced.

t	light tingling	sounds like ligh(t)tingling
d	bad diarrhea	sounds like a ba(d)iarrhea
p	sharp pain	sounds like shar(p)pain
g	a big gash	sounds like a bi(g)gash
k	chronic cough	sounds like croni(c)cough
b	scab bleeding	sounds like scab(b)leeding

Practicing Linking

Take turns describing the symptoms of a client, using phrases from these lists. Try to write two of your own. Link the words together. Use complete sentences.

This client has a sharp pain behind her eyes.
This client has some moles that are infected.

_____

_____

_____

_____

Pronunciation: Intonation in Choice Questions

When you ask a question that has two or more choices, you need to use clear intonation.

<u>Rule</u>: In English, using rising intonation with the first choice and falling intonation with the last choice, if you want the listener to choose one.

Look at the example. Where does intonation rise and fall.

Nursing Assistant: Do you want orange juice (↗) or apple juice (↘)?

Client: O.J., please.

<u>Rule</u>: If your voice only rises at the end of the question, you want the listener to answer with Yes (with a choice) or No (neither choice).

Look at this example.

Nursing Assistant: Do you want something to eat or something to drink (↗)?

Client: No, thanks.

If the meaning is clear, you may ask the question using only the key words.

Nursing Assistant: Orange juice (↗) or apple juice (↘)?

Client: O.J., please.

Using Intonation

Ask each question two ways. First, use a rising and falling intonation pattern. Second, use rising intonation only at the end. Your partner will answer the question appropriately. Imagine the conversations are between two health care workers or between a nurse and a client. Reverse roles.

1. Would you like cream or sugar?

2. Is our next training session on Thursday or Friday?

3. Did you take a bed bath or a shower?

4. Have you been to Memorial or Community General?

5. Does she speak Vietnamese or Tagalog?

6. How about a little water or a little juice?

7. Did you need extra bandages or dressings?

8. Is it better for you to use a cane or a walker?

9. Would it be possible to ask you to either take a nap or go to sleep?

10. Is the surgery scheduled for 9:00 AM or 10:00 AM?

Choosing Appropriate Intonation

Ask these questions only one way. Your partner will answer appropriately based on your intonation. Reverse roles.

1. Did you say fifth floor east or fifth floor west?

2. Does he want to start the treatment or wait a while?

3. Is it O.K. to put your glasses on this tray or on the table?

4. Do you want the shades open or closed?

5. Is your room temperature too hot or too cold?

6. You have two choices: have your husband with you during the birth or be alone.

7. Is the next procedure a rhinoplasty or a liposuction?

8. Would you like it in your I.V. or do you want it in a tablet?

9. Have you received get well cards from your friends or family?

10. Do the residents request more individual activites or group events?

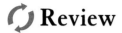# Review

Dialogue Review

Review the dialogue on pages 188–89. As you read, follow the directions. Then compare your answers with a partner.

- Underline the **Symptom** terms.
- Circle the **Discussing the Options** phrase.
- Box the **Advice** phrase.

Role Plays: Symptoms and Remedies

Work with a partner. Read each situation, and develop a dialogue to perform for the class.

1. Two nurses are talking at lunch time. One has a severe earache.

2. Two CNAs are discussing jobs. One wants to know if moving to another hospital is a good idea.

3. An English teacher and a nurse are meeting. The nurse wants to know how to practice English with the clients.

4. Two clients are talking about television programs. They must discuss which one to watch.

5. A nurse and a client are discussing symptoms and remedies. The client wants advice about treating a rash.

6. Two nursing assistants are talking. One wants to know if she should fill the crash cart.

7. A doctor and a client are discussing symptoms. The client is complaining about a severe cough and a continuing backache.

Giving Medications

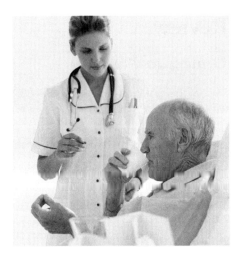

One of the main tasks of many health care workers is to dispense—or give—medication to patients. This must be done carefully. The worker giving the medication must check many details, such as the general description, the medication's purpose, and possible side effects. Health care workers and clients need to focus and get all the information. Sometimes you may have to interrupt to get their attention or get information.

Listening to the Action

Listening for Language

Listen to the conversations. What phrases do the health care workers use to interrupt?

1. _____

2. _____

3. _____

Dialogue

Practicing the Language

A nurse needs to administer medication to a client with an infection. Family and friends are in the room having a conversation with the client. Practice the dialogue in groups of three.

Client: Hey, Austin, tell me about the time you slid off the roof.

Visitor: Well, there I was on the top of the roof. I was balancing on the top, then. . . .

Client: Why were you up there in the first place?

Nurse: [entering the room] May I interrupt for a moment?

Client: Oh, yeah. Hello.

Nurse: Good afternoon, Mr. Ryan. I just need to explain something to you.

Client: O.K. Is it about my new medication?

Nurse: Yes. It's a transdermal morphine patch.

Client: Transdermal means under the skin, right?

Nurse: Actually, it means "through the skin." Your skin will absorb the medication through the surface of your skin.

Visitor: That's right. Hypodermal means "under the skin," like hypodermic needle.

Nurse: That is correct.

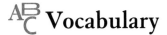 Vocabulary

Symptoms and Remedies

Everyone gets sick sometimes. Health care workers must know how to talk to clients about their symptoms. Specific words will help you understand your client's condition or to better communicate with a doctor.

- **Symptoms**

  Nouns: backache, chest pain, chills, cold, cough, cramps, diarrhea, earache, fever/temperature, headache, infection, rash, runny nose, shortness of breathe, sore throat, stiff neck, stomachache, toothache

  Adjectives: bloated, congested, dizzy, exhausted, itchy, nauseous, swollen

  Verbs: bleeding, sneezing, vomiting, wheezing

- **Remedies** Alka Seltzer™, antacid, antibiotics, aspirin, Band-Aid™, cold medicine, cough medicine, cream, ear drops, heating pad, ice pack, menthol rub, pain killer/reliever, pill/tablet, sleep/rest

Matching Symptoms and Remedies

Match the symptom in the left column with a possible remedy in the right column. Some symptoms could have more than one remedy.

1. rash _____   a. heating pad

2. bloated _____   b. menthol rub

3. infection _____   c. antibiotics

4. stiff neck _____ d. pain killer

5. earache _____   e. cream

6. backache _____   f. Alka Seltzer™

7. sore throat _____ g. cold medicine

8. headache _____   h. ear drops

9. cramps _____   i. throat lozenge

10. sneeze _____   j. aspirin

Using Different Parts of Speech

Complete the table with the correct parts of speech.

Noun	Adjective	Verb
	infectious	infect
	bloody chilly	
	broken	
ache		
congestion		

⇆ Communication Strategy

Correcting Someone

Sometimes the person you are talking to might make a mistake. They might say something untrue or just say it incorrectly. If you need to correct someone, it is important to use polite language. There are many ways to correct someone.

Formal

Actually, it means / I think you mean _____.

Excuse me, but _____.

Sorry, don't you mean _____?

Less formal

Actually _____.

Are you sure?

But _____ is _____, isn't it?

Error Correction

Correct the dialogues about giving or taking medicine. Change the underlined information so it is correct.

1. *Client:*   I need to take my medication <u>before</u> I eat, right?

   Nurse: Actually, I think you mean _____.

2. *Nurse 1:*   TID means they need to take the medication <u>twice a day</u>.

   Nurse 2:   Are you sure? Isn't T.I.D. _____?

3. *Client 1:*   The visiting hours end at <u>9:00 PM</u>.

   Client 2:   Don't you mean _____?

4. *Desk Clerk:*   Did you fill out the section <u>on the bottom</u> about medication allergies?

   Client: But it's _____, isn't it?

5. *Nurse 1:*   The client's tolerance is very high, so we need to give him <u>less</u>.

   Nurse 2:   Sorry, don't you mean _____?

Oral Error Correction

Partners should read their sentences. Then each partner will correct the other.

Partner A

1. You're coughing too much. You need a sedative.

2. Sublingual means talking about someone, right?

3. You will be taking tablets. They're made of plastic.

Partner B

1. Depressants are good for depressed people.

2. Nursing assistants prepare the tranquilizer.

3. I need to take some more antiseptic pills.

Practicing Corrections

Write sentences with wrong information. Read these sentences to a partner. Your partner will correct you. Then reverse roles.

1. _____

2. _____

3. _____

4. _____

5. _____

⇆ Communication Strategy

Interrupting

Often health care workers have to approach a group of people in the middle of a conversation to ask them for information or for help. Or, they are already busy in a group conversation and need to "take the floor" for some reason. There are certain phrases to use, depending on the situation. Proper timing for interruptions is also important. The list of phrases will help get the message across when approaching clients or other health care workers who may be in the middle of a conversation.

Formal

> Excuse me for interrupting, but
> May I interrupt for a moment?
> Please excuse the interruption.

Less Formal

> Excuse me.
> Sorry.

> You can also interject during a conversation.

Formal

> Excuse me for interrupting, but
> I'd like to comment on that.
> I'd like to say something, if I may.
> May I ask something?

Less Formal

> Can I add here that
> Can I add something?
> Can I ask a question?

Sometimes you are interrupted by someone else. If your thought is interrupted, you have to get back to your idea and finish what you were saying. There are phrases to use to signal to the others that you want to continue your speech.

> Anyway,
> Where was I?
> To get back to what I was saying,

Dialogue Practice

Read and practice the dialogues with a small group.

1. *Visitor 1:* . . . and we were sitting there relaxing when we saw it.

   Visitor 2: Yeah, that was funny. When was that again?

   Nurse: Excuse me for interrupting, but it's time for his medication.

   Visitor 1: Oh, is that medication an antibiotic?

   Nurse: Yes it is. Here you go. Sorry for interrupting.

2. *Nurse 1:* So there I was in the OR . . .

   Nurse 2: And? What happened?

   Nursing Assistant: May I interrupt for a moment?

   Nurse 2: Sure.

   Nursing Assistant: The client in 207-A is experiencing breathing problems.

   Nurse 1: O.K. Thank you. I'll check it out now.

Pronunciation: Linking Consonant to Vowel

Part 1 discusses that words ending and beginning with the same consonant are linked.

Listen to your teacher read these phrases. Notice how the words sound.

a dose of	sounds like	a do . . . sof
start an I.V.	sounds like	star . . . ta . . . ni . . . vi
side effect	sounds like	si . . . deffect

Rule: If one word ends with a consonant and the next word begins with a vowel, the two words can link together and sound like one.

Practicing Linking

Read these phrases, and link the words. Work with a partner.

1. swallow it

2. rub it on

3. breathe it in

4. dissolve it

5. inject it

Recognizing Linking

Read the sentences. Underline the places where there is linking with a partner.

1. David's shift ends, and he goes into the locker room.

2. He changes out of his scrubs and into his jeans.

3. He goes out to his car and drives to a restaurant where he meets some friends.

4. He talks about his day and eats a little dinner.

5. The next day, he does it all over again.

Matching

Match the type of mess in the left column with the cleaning method in the right column. Read your answers to a partner, and remember to link consonant to vowel as you say your answer.

1. a pile of cotton swabs that spilled onto the floor _____   a. clean it up

2. a little grease on a cafeteria table _____   b. dust it off

3. urine on the bathroom floor _____   c. mop it up

4. a stain on a washcloth _____   d. rinse it off

5. some mildew in a shower _____   e. scrub it off

6. a fingerprint on the bottom of a glass _____   f. sweep it up

7. some dust on a shelf _____   g. wash it out

8. a pediatric patient's general mess (toys) _____   h. wipe it off

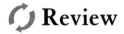 # Review

Dialogue Review

Review the dialogue on page 200. As you read, follow the directions. Then compare your answers with a partner.

- Underline the **Medication** terms.
- Circle the **Correcting** phrase.
- Box the **Interrupting** phrase.

Role Plays: Giving Medications

Work with a partner. Read each situation, and develop a dialogue to perform for the class.

1. A nurse who is new at one hospital needs directions to the laundry room. She interrupts two nurses who are chatting in the break room.

2. A group of student nurses studying for an exam discuss all the ways a medication can enter the body.

3. A nurse is on the phone giving an order to a pharmacist. Another nurse overhears the conversation and corrects the quantity that was ordered.

4. A group of nursing assistants discuss which type of medication (capsules vs. pills and ointments vs. creams) clients prefer.

5. A nurse needs to know the schedule for the next day's operations. She is with some nurses in the cafeteria and interrupts their conversation.

6. A charge nurse is giving orders to an RN for an IM injection. A supervisor is listening and corrects the nurse, saying that it should be an I.V. injection.

7. A client is talking with some visitors. A nursing assistant needs to give the client his medications. She interrupts the conversation.

End-of-Unit Discussion

Sharing

Discuss the questions with a small group.

1. Do you use home remedies? Which kinds do you think are more effective than remedies found in a clinic or hospital? Why?

2. Why do you think it is a good idea to give clients options for their treatment?

3. Do you think some people take too many medications? Explain.

4. What phrases have you used to interrupt a group of people when they are talking? Do you think it is important to use different phrases depending on the group?

Culture Point: Losing Face

Read this story. Discuss in small groups and as a class.

One day a nursing supervisor made a mistake while she was training new nurses about the codes the hospital used. She was explaining Code Rainbow. The chief nursing officer, who was observing the training session, stopped the nursing supervisor and said, "Actually, you mean Code Yellow." The nursing supervisor thanked the chief nursing officer, but the trainees could see that she was upset.

Why was the nursing supervisor upset?

Unit 12: Handling Emotional and Mental Health Issues

Each client has a history and a unique personality. There can be many different reactions to situations when someone is sick or dying. Many times health care workers may experience an angry or violent client or visitor. In these cases, they need to know what kind of communication skills will help keep the situation safe. Other times they may have to deal with a frustrated client who is facing death. It is important to always show empathy and express condolences when death occurs.

Dealing with Angry or Violent Clients

Some clients or their relatives are angry or upset when they are in a medical facility. They may be upset because they don't understand what is happening or they are unhappy about a diagnosis. They may also have other problems like alcohol or drug abuse that cause them to act violently. Some of them just may be tired, emotional, or in pain, so they tend to complain more. Health care workers must be prepared to deal with these situations.

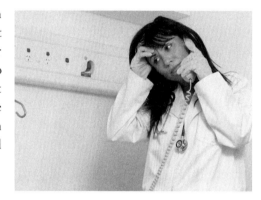

Listening to the Action

Listening for Language

Listen to the conversations between health care workers and angry clients. What phrases do the clients use to complain and which phrases do the health care workers use to respond?

1. _____

2. _____

3. _____

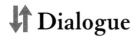 # Dialogue

Practicing the Language

Two nurses are dealing with a client who has become unmanageable. Practice the dialogue in groups of three.

Nurse 1:   We need to try to calm Mr. Kegal down. He still has one hour before the next scheduled morphine drip.

Nurse 2:   I heard he was trying to pull out his catheter tubes and demanded stronger and more frequent doses of his meds.

Nurse 1:   Yes, that's correct. He seems very disobedient. Let's go in and reason with him.

Client: Nurse! This situation is unacceptable. I am in severe pain! These tubes are bothering me, and I need some relief!

Nurse 1:   Mr. Kegal, we are here to help. We need you to take three deep breaths before we can be of assistance.

Client: No way! Don't tell me what to do!

Nurse 2:   Call Security!

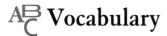 # Vocabulary

Angry or Violent Behavior

It is useful to learn words to describe angry or violent behavior when you are talking to other health care workers. You should not use some of these words when you are charting or reporting an incident. A detailed description of the event and the actions that took place is sufficient.

- **Adjectives:** aggressive, berserk, disgusting, disobedient, disorderly, disruptive, hostile, mad, obnoxious, out of control, stressed, threatening, unmanageable, wild

- **Verbs:** to act violently, to argue, to be defiant, to cause trouble, to curse/swear, to demand, to disturb, to fight

Discussion

Answer the questions with a small group.

1. Which words have similar meanings?

2. Which words should not be used in a formal report? Why not?

Sentence Completion

Complete the sentences with the best word from the lists on page 210. There may be more than one answer. Change the form of the word if necessary.

1. The family members of that client are very _____. Everyone tells them that they must wait in the waiting room, but they keep walking in to the ED.

2. I can't control this guy; he's _____!

3. The parents of the gunshot victim have been a little _____.

4. This teenager wants to fight the nurses. He's acting very _____ now.

5. The trauma unit on Friday and Saturday nights seems to attract the _____ clients.

6. Even though there were no doctors available, the young mother_____ to see a doctor.

7. Mr. Smith's language is strong. He _____ in almost every sentence.

8. Security! We have a man screaming loudly in the lobby. He's _____.

9. That couple can't agree about what to do with their elderly relative. All they do is _____.

10. The little girl with a broken leg is so bored. She thinks it's funny when she _____.

⇆ Communication Strategy

Gestures

You can use your body movements to communicate along with your words. These gestures will help you show that you can follow what is being said and can give clues to your true feelings. Gestures are sometimes understood differently from culture to culture. Some ideas accompanied by gestures in North America are listed. Watch your instructor perform each gesture.

Calm down.
Come here.
Good luck!
I can't hear.
I don't know.
I'm listening.
I'm not listening.
I'm surprised.
No, thank you.

Comparing

Demonstrate the gestures for the ideas in the box on page 211 as you observed or as they are in your native country to a partner.

Determining a Gesture's Meaning

In what kind of situation would you use each of the gestures?

1. Calm down: *a client is angry his dinner is late* _____

2. I don't know: _____

3. Good luck: _____

4. I'm listening: _____

Situation Analysis

Read the situations, and write an appropriate message that could be used. Then add which gesture you could use to accompany the words.

1. A client tells you about his family. _____

2. A family member of a client told you a story about their bad luck with driving a car. They just got into another bad accident. _____

3. A charge nurse gives you an order, but you are not sure what to do. _____

4. Your client will have a big operation tomorrow. _____

5. A client wants to escape from the hospital. _____

6. A client wants to give you money for extra care. _____

7. A supervisor gave you an order from across the room, but you didn't hear. _____

8. You were just hired, but you heard that you might be promoted next month. _____

9. Another nurse is talking about the same thing for the fifth time. _____

10. You need some help and see a certified nursing assistant down the hall. _____

Dialogue Practice

Read and practice the dialogues and gestures with a partner.

1. *Client:* "Let me tell you about my family."

   Nurse: [Gesture for I'm listening.]

2. *Officer:* "Please make sure Mr. Blake gets his prescription ordered."

   Nurse: [Gesture for I don't understand.]

3. *Client:* "I don't want to live anymore! I want to die."

   Nurse: [Gesture for Calm down]

4. *Nurse 1:* "You might have to work overtime tonight!"

   Nurse 2: [Gesture for I'm suprised.]

5. *Client:* "I am going to ask my girlfriend to marry me."

   Nurse: [Gesture for Good luck!]

Matching Other Gestures

Match the statement in the left column with the gestures in the right column. Then practice the gestures with a partner. Check with you instructor.

1. Here I am! _____   a. hang one's head

2. This tastes terrible. _____   b. wave one's arms

3. I feel so ashamed. _____   c. shrug one's shoulders

4. Stop! _____   d. hold one's head up

5. Let me think. _____   e. flag someone down

6. No. _____   f. smile widely

7. I'm not afraid of anything! _____   g. put one's arm around someone

8. Sorry. I don't know. _____   h. stick out one's tongue

9. I am so happy right now! _____   i. shake one's hand

10. I love you. _____   j. scratch one's head

⇆ Communication Strategy

Dealing with Complaints

Part of working with the public is dealing with complaints. Some clients feel that they have the right to complain about various conditions or services in the hospital. Visitors may also do this. Complaints may be direct (which may sound rude) or indirect (which sound polite). There are some phrases that people use when they complain.

Indirect Complaints

Could you please not
I hate to complain, but
I hate to have to say this, but
I'm afraid I'm going to have to complain about
I'm not (exactly) sure how to put this, but
I thought / believe that we had asked you to
Would you mind not

Direct Complaints

I'm tired of dealing with this situation!
I'm very disappointed with this hospital / clinic.
I've had just about enough of this!
This situation is unacceptable.

If you receive a complaint, you need to respond appropriately. In addition to apologizing, you need to assure the client that the problem will be solved. Choose a beginning and an ending.

Complaint Response Beginnings

I apologize for the inconvenience.
I'm very / awfully / terribly / extremely sorry.

Complaint Response Endings

I'll look at it right away.
I'll look into it.
It won't happen again.
We are committed to solving this problem.
We will fix the situation immediately.

Dialogue Practice

Read and practice the dialogues with a partner.

1. *Client:* I hate to have to say this, but you didn't bring me enough medicine.
   Nurse: I'm sorry. I will fix it right away.

2. *Client:* I've had just about enough of this terrible food.
   Nurse: I'm very sorry, Ma'am. What is it about this meal that's bad?

3. *Client:* Would you mind not handling me that way? It's killing my back.
   Nurse: I'm terribly sorry, I will be gentler. It won't happen again.

Complaining

Write a complaint a client could have about each topic.

1. Sharing a room: _____

2. Hospital food: _____

3. Waiting for a doctor: _____

⇆ Communication Strategy

Disagreeing

Sometimes you have a different opinion, idea, or emotion than another person. You can disagree with what he or she says. There are two ways to disagree with someone. The best way to disagree is to disagree formally if possible.

Formal

I hate to disagree with you, but I believe
I respect your opinion, but I think
I understand what you are saying, but in my opinion
I'm not sure if I agree with you.
You could be right, but I don't think that

Less Formal

I may be wrong, but
I'm sorry, but I disagree/don't agree with what you're saying.
That really surprises me because I think

Informal

I don't think so.
Well, I think that
Yes, but

Sometimes you may have to be more direct. Other times it is easier to be direct. With your friends, disagreements can be more direct. Many disagreements are so informal that the conversation may seem funny.

Less Formal

I disagree.
I don't agree.

Informal

Are you joking/kidding!
No way!
That's crazy/absurd/ridiculous!
Uh-uh!
You've got to be joking/kidding!

Dialogue Completion

Complete the dialogue with appropriate phrases from the box on page 216. Then read and practice it with a partner.

Client: I am ready to go home now. I feel wonderful!

Nurse: _____ I believe we have to run a few more tests. You might have to stick around for a couple more days.

Client: because I thought the doctor was finished

Nurse: You can never be too careful, right? Dr. Mullen will be here in the morning. O.K.?

Client: Well, I guess I'm in her hands.

Disagreeing

Read the opinions. Disagree indirectly and directly. Read one or two of your answers to the class.

1. *Client:* In my opinion, I shouldn't be in these wrist restraints.

   Direct: _____

   Indirect: _____

2. *Client:* When a person is sick, the best thing to do is to drink some alcohol because it will help the person get better.

   Direct: _____

   Indirect: _____

3. *Nurse:* It seems that everybody is lazy besides me.

   Direct: _____

   Indirect: _____

Pronunciation: Trimming the Letter *h*

Trimming is when one letter is removed. This happens in reduced speech. Listen to your instructor read the example. What happens to the letter *h*?

| What did he do? | → | What did –e do? |
| Where has he gone? | → | Where –as –e gone? |

Rule: In reduced speech, the letter *h* at the beginning of a pronoun, an adjective, or an auxiliary verb can be silent and linked to the word before it.

Pronouns with "h"	→	he, him, her
Adjectives with "h"	→	his, her
Auxiliary Verbs with "h"	→	has, have, had

Practicing the Silent *h*

Say the phrases using slow speech, and then say them with reduced speech with a partner.

1. What's her . . .
2. should have . . .
3. What had . . .
4. . . . to him.
5. Where had . . .

6. Why has . . .
7. with his . . .
8. Did he . . .
9. about his . . .
10. must have . . .

Recognizing the Silent *h*

Read the sentences. Cross out the letter *h* that should be silent in reduced speech.

1. Help! Let's try to calm him down.
2. We need to give her a sedative.
3. Does he appear to be harmful or just obnoxious?
4. Why has Helen been so violent?
5. Hospital security should have come more quickly.
6. Is his complaint serious? I hope not.
7. We would have heard the code over the loudspeaker.
8. Give him his medication now.

Writing Questions

Write an appropriate question for each answer. Then read the exchanges using reduced speech with a partner.

1. Where _____?

   He went to the O.R.

2. When _____?

   He went at around 10:00 AM.

3. What _____ there?

   He performed an operation.

4. Why _____ do that?

   It was an emergency!

5. Who _____?

   A team of specialists assisted him.

6. How _____ afterwards?

   He felt great!

⟳ Review

Dialogue Review

Review the dialogue on page 210. As you read, follow the directions. Then compare your answers with a partner.

- Underline the **Violent Behavior** terms.
- Circle the **Complaint** phrase.
- Box the **Disagreeing** phrase.

Role Plays: Angry or Violent Clients or Relatives

Work with one or two partners. Read each situation, and develop a dialogue to perform for the class.

1. A family member is using a cell phone in a client's room. A nurse's aide catches him, but he offers a bribe for the aide to be quiet about it.

2. A police officer brings in a suspect who has a gunshot wound to the hand. The suspect starts cursing.

3. Some family members are talking loudly in the waiting area. They are demanding to see a doctor. A nursing assistant tries to calm them.

4. A drug addict in the I.C.U. is trying to leave the bed. A nurse and a security worker are trying to calm him down.

5. An angry relative has come to the nurses' station and is demanding to see a doctor. His child has just died in the ED after a traffic accident.

6. A disorderly woman enters the hospital and says that she is looking for her elderly mother, who is missing from a nursing home. Two workers at the registration desk ask her for some information, but she is not making sense.

7. A thirteen-year-old girl has been hit in the head with a golf club. Her mother brings her to the ED and then begins to behave strangely.

Coping with Death and Dying

Coping with the reality of death may be very difficult for some health care workers. While some clients' deaths are expected, others may die suddenly. Learning to let the person go is part of the training a health care worker receives. Some clients may wish to discuss the issue of death seriously, and others may joke about it. After a client dies, health care workers may need to express their condolences to family members. Sometimes you may not be able to or do not want to answer a question. There are some words to use in these situations.

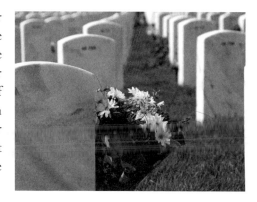

Listening to the Action

Listening for Language

Listen to the conversations. What phrases do the speakers use to express that they cannot answer or will not answer the question?

1. _____

2. _____

3. _____

Dialogue

Practicing the Language

A nurse arrives at the hospital and finds out that her favorite client has died. She talks with her supervisor about it. Practice the dialogue with a partner.

Nurse: I can't believe it. I arrived here at 8:00 and found out that Mrs. Lee passed away overnight. How could that happen? I told her I'd see her tomorrow when I left yesterday.

Supervisor: It's difficult to say, but you knew that she was near the end of her life. We had to let her go.

Nurse: Has her family been here yet?

Supervisor: I've heard that they will stop by soon to pick up her things.

Nurse: What do we say to the family?

Supervisor: Well, just be sincere when you offer condolences. You can say something like, "Please accept my sympathy" or just "I'm sorry."

Nurse: Will the family want to hear about my fun times with their mother?

Supervisor: It depends. We'll see when they get here if they have time to talk.

Nurse: If I miss them, can I get their home phone number?

Supervisor: I'm afraid that's confidential information. Don't worry. I'll make sure that you see them.

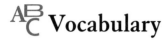 Vocabulary

Near-Death and Death Idioms

It may sound strange, but clients, visitors, or even other health care workers can talk about death by using idioms instead of direct language. There are many idioms used to mean death or dying. Please note that some of them are slang and disrespectful. You may hear them, but shouldn't use them when talking about other people.

- **Near-Death Idioms**

  to be a goner [slang]

  to be about to croak [slang]

  to be about to meet one's maker

  to be at death's door

  to be beyond hope

  to be in a bad way

  to be living on borrowed time

  to be near the end

  to be on one's death bed

  to be on one's last legs

  to be riddled with [cancer]

  to be wasting away

  <u>Note</u>: When talking about a patient who is near death, it's better to add "I'm sorry," "I'm afraid," or "It's so sad" to the sentence to be more respectful.

  I'm sorry to say that she's near the end.

- **Death Idioms**

  to be 6 feet under [slang]

  to be pushing up daisies [slang]

  to go to that great _____* in the sky (slang)

  to kick the bucket [slang]

  to pass

  to pass away / on

* classroom, office, construction site, etc.

Dialogue Completion

Complete these dialogues with an appropriate phrase from the lists on page 222. Then practice with a partner.

1. *Client:*   I'm _____

   Nurse: There's always hope, Mrs. Smith.

2. *Teenager:* My grandmother is going to get better, but my grandfather _____

    _____ (slang)

   Nurse: That's not a nice thing to say.

3. *Relative:*   My brother-in-law is _____, right?

   Nurse: Yes, I'm sorry to say that's true.

Understanding Idioms

Read the sentences and decide if each is disrespectful or acceptable.

1. I heard that your uncle is pushing up daisies. _____

2. He's on his death bed. _____

3. It's very sad, but he's living on borrowed time. _____

4. In 30 years, I'll be pushing up daisies. _____

5. I'm afraid that your father is beyond hope at this time. _____

6. It looks like your sister is going to kick the bucket soon. _____

⇆ Communication Strategy

Avoiding the Issue

Throughout the day you have to answer many questions. Sometimes you either can't or don't want to answer. There are many ways to say "I can't say" (e.g., "I don't know) or "(I know, but) I won't say." When the issue is about the chances of death, it is even more important to not answer directly, as this is the doctor's duty to communicate. These phrases can help you avoid answering.

> How do you mean?
>
> I'd rather not say.
>
> I don't really know.
>
> I have no idea.
>
> I'm afraid that's confidential information.
>
> I'm not in a position to say.
>
> I'm not sure yet.
>
> It depends.
>
> It's difficult to say.
>
> It's hard to tell.
>
> It's not for me to say.
>
> It's too early to say.

Avoiding

Read the phrases in the box. Underline the ones that mean "I can't say," and circle the ones that mean "I won't say."

Dialogue Practice

Read and practice the dialogues with a partner.

1. *Client:*   Are you going to increase my dosage? I told you, I need more!

   Nurse: I don't really know. I will ask the doctor for you.

2. *Client:*   Do you think I will die soon?

   Nurse: I'm not really in a position to say.

3. *Nurse 1:*   How much does our supervisor earn?

   Nurse 2:   I'm afraid that is confidential information.

   Nurse 1:   Oh, I'm sorry. This is open information in my culture.

Dialogue Completion

Complete the dialogues with an appropriate avoidance phrase from the box on page 224.

1. *Nurse 1:*   Does Nurse Makiko want you to cover her shift?

   Nurse 2: _____.

2. *Client:*   How much money does my doctor make?

   Nurse: _____.

3. *Head Nurse:*   Where is the schedule? I don't see it.

   Nurse: _____.

4. *Client:*   Why didn't you call last night?

   Visitor: _____.

5. *Visitor:*   Tell me the truth. Is my father's situation beyond hope?

   Nurse: _____.

⇆ Communication Strategy

Expressing Condolences

No matter where you work in the health care industry, you will either hear about a death or experience it directly. As this is a difficult time for family and friends, it may be comforting to them if you express condolences. Note the difference between condolences for deaths that happen where you work and those that you hear about (that happened in a different place or in the past).

Formal

I am so/very sorry for your loss.
I am so/very sorry to hear of your loss.
Please accept my sympathy/condolences.
You have my (deepest) sympathy/condolences.

Less Formal

I'm so/very sorry.
I'm sorry.
I'm sorry to hear about [person's name].
I'm sorry to hear about your [relative].

Writing Condolences

Choose an appropriate condolence phrase from the box on page 225 to use in each situation.

1. You are in the room when a doctor has just told a client's husband that his wife has died in the ED.

   _____.

2. You hear that one client's brother has died. That client comes to her appointment at the doctor's office.

   _____.

3. The family of a client who has died after a long illness comes to the hospital to thank the nurses for all that they did.

   _____.

4. A client has told you that her 12-year-old dog has just died (since she has been in the hospital).

   _____.

5. Someone tells you that a co-worker was out yesterday to attend the funeral of her grand-mother. The co-worker returns to work.

   _____.

6. You are chatting with a relative of one of your clients. This person tells you about several people in the family who have died this year.

   _____.

Situation Analysis

Read the situations and the condolences. Mark the condolence that is inappropriate. Then talk with a partner about your choices.

1. A young boy dies of leukemia. A nurse who took care of the client every day talks to the parents.

   _____ Condolence 1: Please accept my sympathy, Mr. and Mrs. Jones. Billy was a fighter to the end.

   _____ Condolence 2: I'm sorry to hear about your son, Mr. and Mrs. Jones.

2. A respiratory therapist tells a co-worker that his grandfather passed away.

   _____ Condolence 1: That's too bad. These things happen to old people.

   _____ Condolence 2: I'm sorry for your loss.

3. A client tells a nursing assistant that her husband died 20 years ago from a heart attack.

   _____ Condolence 1: You have my deepest sympathy. You must be very sad. I'm sorry for your loss.

   _____ Condolence 2: Oh, I'm sorry.

Pronunciation: Contractions

Your native language may or may not have contractions, but they are very common in oral English. Most contractions may also be written.

Making Contractions

Complete the chart with the correct contraction of the verbs and modals in the top row combined with the words in the left column. Some have been filled in for you. Some boxes in the last column will be blank.

	am/is/are	will	would	have/has
I				I've
You				
He		He'll		
She				
It			It'd	
We				
They				
There	There's/There're			
That				

Practicing Contractions

Read each situation, and choose an appropriate phrase to say.

It'll be O.K. to cry at the funeral.   That's been confidential for years.

He's wasting away.   There'll be happier times.

I'd rather not give an opinion.   They've passed on.

1. A woman talking about her grandparents.

   _____

2. Someone who is speaking to a deceased client's relatives at a memorial service.

   _____

3. A nurse who has been asked who the best doctor in the hospital is.

   _____

4. A mother talking to her children before going to a funeral.

   _____

5. A hospital president talking about releasing clients' social security numbers.

   _____

6. A woman who is sad about her husband's condition.

   _____

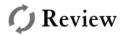 Review

Dialogue Review

Review the dialogue on page 221. As you read, follow the directions. Then compare your answers with a partner.

- Underline the **Near-Death and Death** terms.
- Circle the **Avoid the Issue** phrases.
- Box the **Condolence** phrases.

Role Plays: Death and Dying

Work with a partner. Read each situation, and develop a dialogue to perform for the class.

1. A very ill client is talking with a relative. She uses some idioms to express that she will soon die. The relative tries to encourage her.

2. A client's relative has heard a rumor that the hospital is in trouble and will close. He asks a nurse about this, but she isn't permitted to say anything.

3. A supervisor asks a nursing assistant about some supplies that are missing. The nursing assistant doesn't know anything about them

4. A nurse expresses her condolences to a co-worker whose father just died.

5. A nursing assistant hears a teenager use some death and dying idioms about residents in his grandmother's nursing home. She teaches him some more acceptable phrases.

6. A nurse comforts the wife of a client who has just died in the trauma center.

7. A client who had quadruple bypass surgery asks a nurse if he will be able to eat anything he wants soon after he's discharged. A nurse explains that the doctor will be able to answer the question.

End-of-Unit Discussion

Sharing

Discuss the questions with a small group.

1. How does the anger of a client or a client's relative hurt the healing process?

2. Which gesture(s) do you use the most? Which new gestures from this unit have you tried? What was the other person's reaction?

3. Compared to your culture, do health care workers where you work give out more information or less information to the client's family?

4. What are some ways to not be too emotionally affected by a client's death?

Culture Point: Confusion with Idioms

Read this story. Discuss in small groups and as a class.

The nurses and hospital staff were prepping one of the clients, Ron, for his surgery scheduled for later in the day. Ron liked to joke with the nurses, and he was in a good mood. Ron's doctor stopped by the room to greet Ron and asked him if he had any last-minute questions about the surgery.

Ron: Yes, doctor. I have a question. Will I be pushing up daisies after the surgery?

Doctor: Well . . . sure, Mr. Croteau! You will be pushing up lots of daisies soon after the surgery. Ha Ha! See you soon.

The doctor left the room. Ron looked very worried. Why?

Culture Point Explanations

Unit 1 Culture Point (page 22)

Possible answer:

Mr. Vong is from a culture where a smile can mean many things, including an apology. Gabrielle thinks that Mr. Vong smiled because he did not care about what she had been teaching him and that he did not understand how important the injections were. Until someone tells Gabrielle what a smile can mean, she will misinterpret some clients' reactions.

Unit 2 Culture Point (page 38)

Possible answer:

The man and his wife is from a culture in which child care is basically a woman's job. When the children become teenagers, men have a more important role. The husband was happy that his daughter was being discharged, but did not want to hear any details about her care at home since he would not be involved.

Unit 3 Culture Point (page 58)

Possible answer:

Physical contact (hugging and kissing) with people you have just met is not normal in the United States. The student is from a culture where hugs and even kisses are normally used in introductions and greetings. The student's parents were so relieved that their daughter was recovering that the hugs were meant to show their appreciation. This had never happened to the head nurse before. The student quickly explained proper greeting customs to her parents.

Unit 4 Culture Point (page 79)

Possible answer:

Satoko is from a culture in which it is very difficult to say no. In her culture, people would know that *Maybe* meant no, especially since she didn't give any explanation. She said *O.K.* only to indicate to Amber that she understood what she wanted. Satoko takes the bus and doesn't want to get involved in the protest.

Unit 5 Culture Point (page 98)

Possible answer:

Priva is from a culture in which workers feel better and more productive if they work under close supervision from a supervisor. She wasn't used to having freedom on the job. She would have felt more comfortable if the actual supervisor were around to train her in her new position.

Unit 6 Culture Point (page 117)

Possible answer:

The supervisor saw that Bandhi's work was excellent and he drew a conclusion about Bandhi's future. Yolanda gave a normal American reaction to good news. Bandhi is from a culture where the future cannot be so highly predictable. Fate may cause many things to change. Instead of transferring to better jobs, something bad may happen and he may be laid off or let go. He feels safer dealing with the present than thinking about the future and what may happen years from now.

Unit 7 Culture Point (page 138)

Possible answer:

Rachel was insulted when Debra said, "Don't be crazy." She knew that the word *crazy* meant mentally ill, and she didn't want her supervisor to think that she was mentally ill. According to her culture, she was also worried that Debra thought she was slow and incompetent because she couldn't finish her tasks during her shift. Another CNA who saw what happened explained to Rachel that in the United States it's perfectly acceptable to accept help and that during a shift change to tell the oncoming nurses what still needs to be done.

Unit 8 Culture Point (page 152)

Possible answer:

The CNAs are from a culture where the supervisors, if they really like the work, take time to give lavish praise. A small amount of praise may sound like a small criticism instead. They need to learn that in the United States, simple and direct praise is normal.

Unit 9 Culture Point (page 168)

Possible answer:

Melanie is from a culture where it is embarrassing to be singled out. It is fine if her entire department is praised, but for Melanie to be named the Employee of the Month might mean that her peers could react negatively. Fortunately, Melanie was told that this procedure is normal in U.S. culture, and she accepted the honor.

Unit 10 Culture Point (page 187)

Possible answer:

Mrs. Aoki obviously didn't speak English well enough to even understand Nurse Victoria's question. It was easier for her to just say yes. Also, she is from a culture where it is embarrassing to say no, so she tends to say yes to appear more cooperative. She thought that later on she would find out from somebody if she were doing it wrong.

Unit 11 Culture Point (page 208)

Possible answer:

The nursing supervisor most likely lost face when she was corrected in front of the new nurses. In her culture, any supervisor would have told her privately about her mistake, and then let her tell the nurses the correct information in her own way. It was embarrassing and upsetting to be corrected like that in front of those she was training.

Unit 12 Culture Point (page 230)

Possible answer:

The doctor was a non-native English speaker and had never heard of the idiom *to be pushing up daisies*. He would never imagine that a client would make a joke about dying. He assumed that *pushing up daisies* meant that Mr. Croteau would be able to enjoy his garden again. After one of the nurses explained to both Ron and the doctor the misunderstanding, Ron felt better.